THIS WON'T HURT

(And Other Lies My Doctor Tells Me)

THIS WON'T HURT

(And Other Lies My Doctor Tells Me)

*Observations From
the Other End of the Stethoscope*

By Charles B. Inlander
President, People's Medical Society

≡People's Medical Society®
Allentown, Pennsylvania

The People's Medical Society is a nonprofit consumer health organization dedicated to the principles of better, more responsive and less expensive medical care. Organized in 1983, the People's Medical Society puts previously unavailable medical information into the hands of consumers so that they can make informed decisions about their own health care.

Membership in the People's Medical Society is $20 a year and includes a subscription to the *People's Medical Society Newsletter.* For information, write to the People's Medical Society, 462 Walnut Street, Allentown, PA 18102, or call 610-770-1670.

Library of Congress Cataloging-in-Publication Data

Inlander, Charles B.
    This won't hurt (and other lies my doctor tells me) : observations from the other end of the stethoscope / by Charles B. Inlander.
        p.   cm.
    ISBN 1-882606-39-6
    1. Medical care. 2. Consumer education. 3. Patient satisfaction.
    4. Medical policy. 5. Medical personnel and patient. I. Title.
    R727.I54 1998
    362.1—dc21   98-13883
                                                                      CIP

1 2 3 4 5 6 7 8 9 0

First printing, June 1998

The information in this book is intended to help the reader make more informed choices regarding health care. It is not a substitute for expert medical advice or treatment. All matters regarding health require medical supervision.

Many of the designations used by manufacturers and sellers to distinguish their products are claimed as trademarks. Where those designations appear in this book and People's Medical Society was aware of a trademark claim, the designations have been printed in initial capital letters (e.g., Band-Aid).

We have tried to use male and female pronouns in an egalitarian manner throughout the book. Any imbalance is in the interest of readability.

CONTENTS

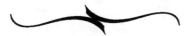

PREFACE

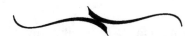

This Won't Hurt!

When I was a kid growing up in Chicago, I hated going to the doctor. My pediatrician was a nice enough man. He always seemed kind, and he would always tell me jokes. I didn't mind his office, either. The receptionist was very friendly. There were plenty of magazines for kids lying around. And there were even some toys to tinker with while I waited.

But the one thing that really bothered me about him was that he lied. And the worst part about his lying was that he thought he was doing it for my own good. I know he lied to all my friends, as well. When I told them about the lies he told me, they would say he told them the same thing. As a result, I developed a great mistrust of doctors.

Of course, the biggest lie he told was when he would say, "This won't hurt, Charles!" and then proceed to give me a painful shot. He joked that he practiced his shots on grapefruits—he even had a hypodermic needle sticking out of a wooden replica of a grapefruit on his desk. But he only chuckled when I reminded him that wooden things had no feelings.

Granted, shots are not all that painful, but most kids think they are. And when a doctor tries to ease a child into one by saying it won't hurt—and the child knows otherwise—well, it's not hard to figure out why a kid might hate going to the doctor.

Over the years, doctors have lied to me repeatedly. Sometimes, it was about pain. I remember my first rectal exam when the doctor wanted to check my prostate gland. His exact words were, "This may bother you a little, but it won't hurt too much." Frankly, I thought his hand was going to reach my throat, the pain was so severe. Other times, the lies were more subtle and serious. I once had a doctor tell me that he had performed a certain diagnostic test many times, but I later found out that I was the first patient on whom he'd done the procedure. I never used him again.

I've received tens of thousands of letters from consumers since we started the People's Medical Society in 1983. And one of the consistent themes is mistrust of doctors. People complain about not being told the truth about their conditions. Consumers scream when they see bills submitted to insurers for services never rendered. They are indignant with medical professionals who ignore living wills and perform unwanted services on dying family members.

There is an arrogance about medicine that seems to have infiltrated the behavior of far too many medical professionals. And believe me, this is not just limited to doctors. There is nothing more frustrating than being confined to a hospital bed and not being able to get a nurse to respond to repeated pushes of the call button. And why should a consumer—in reality a customer—have to fight with a hospital administrator just to get an itemized bill for a $20,000 hospital stay? Is there anything more irritating than being endlessly left on hold, listening to canned music, when you're trying to get an answer to an insurance problem only to find that the "account executive" you eventually reach knows less than you do?

These are not easy times for health care consumers. Forty-three million Americans are without health insurance.

In some communities, up to 50 percent of children arrive at first grade without their required immunizations. Nationally, more than half the hospital beds are empty, and more and more not-for-profit hospitals are merging or selling out to for-profit chains. Managed care has become the dominant trend in medical care and insurance, shifting the power away from practitioners and putting it into the hands of large insurance companies. Medicare and Medicaid are being reviewed and revised, bringing fundamental changes to both programs. And with every change, with each new trend, consumers are left out in the cold. At the same time, reports of fraud within the health care system are becoming commonplace.

Today, health care is the largest industry in America! It employs more people than any other type of business. It consumes more of the gross domestic product than any other segment of the economy. And it serves more customers than ever before. Yet it is the last bastion of nonconsumerism in this country. We still get less information about doctors, hospitals and drugs than we do about any other consumer service or product. And what is even more troublesome, consumers are very rarely invited to participate in helping to make the system more responsive and consumer oriented.

Think about it. Rarely are consumer voices heard commenting on the major issues influencing their health and medical care. And even when they are heard, the voice is usually that of a victim of the medical system. We hear the man who had the wrong leg removed during a hospital procedure. We listen to the husband whose wife died when physicians operated on the wrong side of her brain. We have the writings of a health reporter who died from an overdose of an experimental medication for breast cancer.

These cases, as compelling and newsworthy as they are, tend to be the only kind that bring consumers into the health care debate. As victims, consumers make news. They can increase the ratings on *Dateline NBC* and *60 Minutes.* They provide faces and fodder for congressional hearings on proposed legislation. But more often, medical consumers are talked about but never invited to speak. In other words, the voice of health care consumerism has not been taken seriously by policy makers and providers of care.

The typical health care consumer is confused about the changes going on in medical care. Is managed care beneficial? Are hospital mergers in our best interests? Have nursing homes and long-term-care facilities improved in recent years? Is my doctor obsolete? What about pharmacists—are there better ways to distribute medications? Do I have rights as a medical consumer? In this electronic age, is my medical privacy being compromised? How qualified is my doctor? Should I worry that my local hospital is shutting down? Questions such as these are on all our minds. And answers are few.

In addition, the medical marketplace is getting muddled. For the first time in American medical history, consumers are being forced to leave their current doctors in favor of those chosen by their insurers or employers. People are being denied admission to hospitals that do not contract with certain insurers. Doctors are discharging patients from hospitals based on orders of insurance companies, rather than on medical readiness.

Consumers are angry and upset. A July 1996 Harris poll reported that health care is the second highest concern among consumers, trailing only crime as an issue. Most members of Congress report that health care issues rank first, on a year-to-year basis, in the mail they receive.

And while consumers write letters to the editors of their local newspapers and complain to one another about the state of health care in the United States, there has been very little public venting of people's concerns and worries. And the public's anxiety is increasing. In 1997, for the first time, most managed care companies began having financial problems. Consumers began to worry about the long-term viability of their plans. Many Medicare health maintenance organizations announced cutbacks in the extra benefits often provided to lure elderly folks into their programs.

The American health care system seems to have very little regard for the people it serves. What was once a profession of caring and compassion has become an industry of greed and deceit, involving everything from lying to patients to submitting bills for services not rendered. Even the good people (and there are many) who practice medicine, work in hospitals or provide other services related to health care have been sucked into this abyss of lies and arrogance, not by what they do, but by not doing anything about the abuse they see around them. It's sad that those who know better are afraid to speak out. And yet, in some ways, I can understand why. Let me relate an experience that might make the point more vivid.

Back in the mid-1980s, a newspaper was preparing a feature article on the People's Medical Society and me. Back then, medical consumerism was a new concept. Doctors and hospitals were outraged that someone like me, a nonphysician, was challenging those in the health care system to be more responsive to consumers. Our book *Take This Book to the Hospital With You* had been out about a year and was a best-seller. I had been on all the major television shows from *Oprah* to *Today*. So it was natural that this newspaper wanted to find out more about me and the organization.

I did an extensive interview with the reporter. We talked about my background in consumer advocacy, the history of the People's Medical Society and our goals for the future. A few days before the article was to run, the reporter called me. "Mr. Inlander," he said, "we have a problem." I wasn't sure what he meant.

He proceeded to tell me that his editor had asked him to talk to doctors about their reactions to the People's Medical Society and, specifically, to me. He did talk to a number of doctors, including the then president of the American Medical Association. All of them had strong opinions about the organization. Several questioned the need for an organization of medical consumers—doctors are consumer advocates, they claimed.

But one doctor raised some serious questions. The fellow was a practitioner who practiced in the community where the People's Medical Society was headquartered. He didn't like the organization from the day it was founded. On several occasions, he had confronted me personally, challenging my "credentials" to do what I was doing. Of course, I didn't know I needed credentials to work for consumer rights, but this physician just didn't like the idea that a layperson would take on the world of medicine.

The reporter was upset when he talked to me. It seems that this doctor had told the reporter that I was a demagogue who was only doing what I did for self-promotion. He went on to tell the reporter that he knew exactly why I was so "antidoctor." He said that I was jealous of my older brother who had become a doctor. He went on to say that I had been turned down by medical schools and that I had gotten involved with this work because of my jealousy and rage.

The reporter asked me for my reaction. I very calmly told the reporter to run the story and include the information provided by the doctor. I asked him to be sure, however, to identify the doctor in the story.

The reporter was surprised. "Are you sure you want us to run that? My editor asked me to call you and discuss it."

"Run it!" I laughed.

"What's so funny?" he wanted to know.

"Well, the fact is," I began, "I don't have a brother. I'm an only child. Second, I've never applied to a medical school. Being a doctor is the last thing I have aspired to be. And third, I can't wait to sue the bastard for slander once his words are published!"

Needless to say, the doctor's comments did not appear in the story. I even had a call from the managing editor of the paper, who was appalled at the lies this doctor had tried to get published in the paper.

But frankly, I wasn't surprised. Because, as I noted earlier, lying and medicine have become synonymous.

So here I sit in 1998, as outraged as ever about the American health care system. And that is exactly why I have written this book. I'm angry. I'm mad that those in power are doing too little to help the health care consumer. I'm irritated that medical professionals, hospital personnel, insurance companies and politicians are not listening to the voices of their customers and their constituents.

So what follows are my views about today's health care scene. These are observations from the other end of the stethoscope—the round, cold end. My intention is to do more than vent. I hope that these observations spark your thinking and maybe even motivate you to take action. If you're a health care consumer (and we all are!), I hope my comments empower you to be more proactive in your health care. I also hope these essays motivate you to speak out about health care issues. The more we, as consumers, make our voices heard in the highest places on these issues, the more likely changes are to occur.

But I am not just directing my views to consumers. I also want medical professionals and health care policy makers to realize that consumers can no longer be ignored. We are more than just conditions and cash flow—we are the reason the health care industry exists. We have tolerated too many indignities and too much shoddy care to allow our views and voices to be ignored.

Acknowledgments

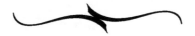

Many people have helped me create this book. At the People's Medical Society, Janet Worsley Norwood served as the project manager and primary editor. Her comments, enthusiasm and direction have been both invaluable and motivating. I appreciate her important input. Jennifer Hay also served as an important editor helping me refine and hone my words. She deserves many thanks. Jerry O'Brien designed the book and, as always, did a great job. And thanks, too, to Linda Hager and Sue Kittek for their detailed and extremely helpful editing.

A very special thanks to Madge Kaplan, health desk editor for Public Radio International's *Marketplace*. Many of the observations found in this book are built from commentaries I have made as a health commentator on *Marketplace*. Madge is a fantastic editor who has helped me say what I want to say in a much better way. I am forever grateful for her assistance.

Lowell Levin, professor of public health at Yale University and former chairperson of the People's Medical Society, has been both my mentor and inspiration for more than 15 years. Lowell's commitment to medical consumerism and his fearless advocacy of issues, often unpopular with his colleagues, have motivated me to continue speaking out even when the darts are being thrown.

Finally, I want to thank the tens of thousands of consumers who have supported the People's Medical Society and me since the early 1980s. Without that support, the voice of medical consumers would be virtually unheard.

PART I

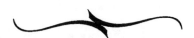

Angry, Enraged, Furious, Incensed, Infuriated, Irate, Mad, Seething— *You've Gotta Know How I Feel!*

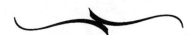

OK, so maybe I am emotional. But I know you share my feelings. I mean, look, I've had tens of thousands of letters from health care consumers over the years, and the words above have been in most of those letters. Let's face it—most of us are just plain fed up with the way we're treated by medical practitioners and facilities, not to mention the politicians and policy makers who dabble in health care.

This first section of the book is a bit of venting. But believe me, I am not just blowing off steam. The issues I discuss here are the reasons we have to be vigilant medical consumers. And I know there are many other matters that irk you that I do not discuss. But don't be dismayed. The important thing is that we're all getting angry. That means we're catching on to what's going on, and then maybe we'll unite to do something about it.

You're
a Jerk

"Charles Inlander, you're a jerk."

That was the one-sentence letter I received from a doctor who disagreed with my position on medical malpractice.

If you believe the doctor's side of the argument, you would think that doctors are heading to the poorhouse due to malpractice suits. It's just not true. Overall, malpractice premiums—the fees doctors pay for malpractice insurance—have remained steady or gone down over the last 10 years. The number of lawsuits has actually declined, as has the average payment to victims. In fact, all the costs associated with medical malpractice, from premiums to payouts, add up to less than 2 percent of the nation's total expenditure on health care.

Malpractice rates, however, haven't declined. Back in 1991, a Harvard study found that 86,000 people die each year from hospital negligence. In February 1997, a study reported in the prestigious medical journal *Lancet* suggested that the number of unnecessary hospital deaths may be three times that estimated in the Harvard study.

However, the Harvard study said, only 1 percent of malpractice victims ever file a claim, and more than 70 percent of those who do file lose their cases, in part because doctors are reluctant to testify against colleagues.

But physicians continue to lobby to change malpractice laws. They want to limit the ability of injured consumers to get access to the courthouse and, short of that, cap the amount of money judges or juries can award. And of course, they never tell you the other side of the story.

I'm a jerk simply because I talk publicly about these issues.

Actually, what I really am is a health care consumer. Maybe I'm a bit more daring than the typical user of health services. And I probably have a bigger mouth than most other people. But I believe that medical care is a service. I purchase the care; someone else delivers it. As a customer, I expect respect, a high-quality product and accountability. Sadly, most Americans do not get all three—and many get none.

Health care remains the last bastion of nonconsumerism in America. We receive less information about our doctors, hospitals and health insurance providers than we do about bank loans or funeral services. Think about it: When a person applies for a mortgage, the lender is required to disclose all the terms, including interest rates, penalties for early payoffs and what actions either the lender or the borrower can take if something goes wrong. When a funeral is being planned, the funeral director is required to make disclosures. All costs must be in writing. Services are described, and payment options are explained.

But no similar disclosure is required by doctors, hospitals or even managed care companies. For example, no state requires a doctor to routinely disclose to a patient his training, the number of times he has performed a procedure, his outcome rates on certain procedures—such as the number of deaths or of patients with complications—or the number of lawsuits he has lost or settled.

Health care consumers are expected to choose, use and pay for medical care based on blind faith, without having the information necessary to make informed decisions. We are expected to assume that all doctors are equally competent or qualified. We are supposed to accept that every hospital is as good as the next one. And we are supposed to trust managed care plans such as health maintenance organizations when they advertise that they choose only the best doctors.

In other words, when it comes to health care, we're treated like children—very tiny ones, at that. It is presumed by those in the health care system that we, as consumers, are not bright enough to understand our conditions, the differences between doctors or the quality of hospitals. We're medical idiots—simply because we have not gone through the terror of medical school. And if we challenge the system, we are called "jerk" or are presumed to have a mental illness.

The entire medical system is designed to intimidate the consumer. Most doctors like to call their patients by their first names but prefer to be called "doctor" when being addressed. That's astounding! When I use any other service, the provider calls me "Mr. Inlander." Only after I say it's OK will I be called by my first name.

Even the language of medicine is anticonsumer in its intimidating nature. Why can't doctors simply say a person had a "heart attack" instead of a "myocardial infarction"? My mechanic tells me that my fuel line is clogged, not that the injectors are impregnated with obstacles. While over-the-counter medications are rather simply named, prescription drugs carry complicated monikers even many doctors cannot pronounce.

And why do so many states make special "M.D." license

plates for physicians to put on their cars? I see more of them in parking lots of fancy restaurants on Saturday nights than I do at hospitals on weekday mornings. And who invented the notorious hospital gown? If you know what asylum that designer has been committed to, I'd like the address.

Most consumers are just not taken seriously by health care professionals. Studies show that consumers get an average of 18 seconds to explain their problem to a physician before being interrupted. And there is nothing worse than having to sit around a doctor's waiting room with coughing, gagging and sniffling copatients while the doctor sees "an emergency." Well, maybe there is something worse—having to wait 15, 30 or even 60 minutes after the assigned appointment time to be seen. I really cheered a few years ago when a Florida man sued his doctor for keeping him waiting. He won! The court said the patient's time was just as valuable as the doctor's.

Maybe I'm crazy, but I was raised to believe that health care was meant to serve those in need. But our health care system has historically been set up to serve the providers of care. This is especially true of hospitals. From the lobby to the patient care room, hospitals are about the last place in the world one would choose to go to heal or have an illness treated.

One problem is the noise. Have you ever noticed how loud hospitals are? Outside, there are signs that say "Quiet—Hospital Zone." Inside, it sounds like the north-south runway of Chicago's O'Hare Airport.

Loudspeaker announcements are blaring night and day. Doctors and nurses are talking right outside patients' rooms at all hours of the night. Televisions blast, machinery whirs, and visitors yuk it up while most patients are trying to sleep or rest. About a decade ago, a study found the decibel levels at most large hospitals were so high they actually slowed down patient recovery time.

But that's not all that's anticonsumer about hospitals. These days, because more than half the hospital beds in the country are empty, institutions have launched advertising campaigns as a way to attract customers. My favorite ads are the ones that claim "We Care" or "Compassion Is What Sets Us Apart." Talk about the lack of truth in advertising! If these facilities really cared or were so compassionate, why would patients say it takes several minutes or more for a nurse to respond when the call button is pushed? Or how about the studies that show hospitals are cutting back on highly trained registered nurses and substituting minimally trained aides, claiming at the same time that care is not affected? Poppycock!

By now you probably think that I hate doctors and hospitals—but let me assure you that isn't true. There are many fine physicians and outstanding hospitals. But most consumers have no means of knowing who and where those are. The vast majority of us go from doctor to doctor, hospital to hospital or health service to health service knowing nothing about their quality. And that's just no longer acceptable.

The health care system in this country must become accountable. Any person using a health provider or service should be able to find out how well practitioners practice or how effective a hospital is in providing care. Information about outcomes must replace fluffy ads and airy billboards.

Medical leaders, insurance providers and politicians alike

must recognize that we are not medical idiots. We want high-quality services, useful and relevant information and accountability from those who serve us.

But most important, we want a health care system that is responsive to our needs as consumers. And until we get it, more and more of us will become jerks. And nobody likes a jerk!

Clueing
Us In

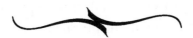

Would you go to a doctor who lost or settled 33 medical malpractice cases in a two-year period? Thousands of Michigan residents did. Or how about a physician who had more than 300 charges brought against him by a state medical licensing board? His practice flourished in Pennsylvania. Would you make an appointment with a physician whose local medical society believed he was a threat to public safety? For years after that indictment, Ohio women kept pouring into his office.

How could these people be so dumb? Why would they go to such dreadful practitioners? The answer is simple—they didn't know their practitioners' records. And what's worse, they had no way of finding out.

In all three of these cases, the medical licensing board— the state agency responsible for protecting consumers from bad doctors—wouldn't reveal the damaging information. If that sounds strange, think again. All across the country, these agencies have a history of protecting practitioners rather than the public.

That is beginning to change, and none too soon. In November 1996, Massachusetts led the way by passing legislation that made public the information the state holds about doctors. Consumers can now call in and find out about a doctor's education, specialty certification, hospital practice privileges and any criminal, malpractice and medical board disciplinary actions.

More states are jumping on the bandwagon. In Florida, the licensing board has agreed in principle that the public has the right to know about physicians who have multiple malpractice claims filed against them. And another Florida agency is seeking legislation to be allowed to release more information about physicians and hospitals.

In Pennsylvania, several legislators have introduced a bill similar to the Massachusetts law that would make public physicians' professional records.

In Washington State, an even more revealing piece of legislation is being considered. Introduced by the state's department of health, the proposal would make public even complaints that are being investigated. This is truly a revolutionary proposal. Today, not one state even tells the consumer who filed a complaint what its investigators uncovered.

Frankly, it's about time the door to physician competence was pried open. For too long, the foxes have been guarding the chicken coop as physicians' trade associations have used their money and influence to keep the public at bay. Now consumers are beginning to get the information necessary to make informed choices about practitioners. And states are recognizing that they have an obligation to protect consumers from shoddy medical practice.

I know many of the victims of the three doctors I mentioned earlier. If there had been laws like those we've discussed in place in their states, very few of them would be suffering today from the disfigurement, infertility or pain that they have. And while it's too late for them, it's not too late for the rest of us.

A panel appointed by President Clinton to establish a "bill of rights" for consumers in managed care plans released its recommendations in late 1997. Among them were proposals demanding more disclosure about the physicians contracted by the plans. It remains to be seen if these proposals will be adopted by the managed care industry or passed into law by the federal and state governments. But it is clear that consumers want practitioners and health plans to be held accountable. And that can happen by making a doctor's record—and both the good and the bad in it—public.

Even the American Medical Association is making an attempt to get into the act. In November 1997, it announced its own program to accredit physicians. The idea here, in a nutshell, is that the AMA checks out doctors against a set of standards it has devised and accredits those who meet the standards. A lot of what it has found will not be made public, but health maintenance organizations and other managed care companies can purchase this information, including the nonpublic findings, rather than having to check out a doctor on their own. It remains to be seen if this will be successful or not. I mean, one can hardly trust a trade association such as the AMA to be working hard for consumers when its dues-paying constituency is made up of doctors. But at least it's an acknowledgment that times are changing. Public demand is winning out.

Even with the AMA's program and the federal panel's recommendation, it's important to remember that health care is still regulated at the state level. Only states license doctors. Only states can discipline substandard ones. So it is clearly, first and foremost, a state's job to assure the public of the competence of those it licenses.

In this day and age, there is no justification for any state government to keep bad news about doctors away from the public. And the quicker every state legislature understands that, the better it will be for us all.

Woman as a Disease

American medicine has made the word *woman* a medical diagnosis. You won't find it defined that way in the dictionary. Lexicographers still insist it merely means an adult female human being. But in the eyes of many in the medical profession, womanhood is a disease just waiting to be treated.

Over the last 30 years, the biggest medical scandals have been perpetrated on women. It was women who were prescribed the dangers of diethylstilbestrol, thalidomide, the Dalkon Shield and silicone breast implants. Nothing comparable has happened to men.

But that's not all. Women are far more likely to be cut open than men. Consider the hysterectomy: surgery to remove the uterus. In 1998, more than 550,000 will be performed. Medical experts conservatively say that at least half of all hysterectomies are unnecessary.

And there are other curious trends. The rate of hysterectomy in the southern United States is almost double that of any other region in the country. And there are more hysterectomies performed in communities that have lots of doctors and hospitals—places such as wealthy suburbs.

Money has a lot to do with it. Statistics show that doctors are far less likely to recommend a hysterectomy to an uninsured woman than to one with a high-option insurance plan from her employer.

Here's another example: cesarean sections. The c-section rate went from 5 percent in 1970 to 24 percent in 1997. More than 900,000 c-sections were performed in 1997. It's the most performed operation in American hospitals. Yet it hasn't increased a woman's chances of surviving childbirth, and it hasn't improved infant mortality rates. Could it be that baby-boomer mothers are anatomically inferior to their own mothers who had far fewer c-sections? You're right—that's preposterous! Has the nearly 500 percent increase in the number of cesareans performed occurred because doctors fear lawsuits due to botched births? Sure, the number of these lawsuits has doubled in the last 25 years, but so has the number of ob-gyns. In other words, the increase in the number of lawsuits is proportional to the number of ob-gyns, not to a lawsuit-happy public. Do you ever wonder why the c-section rates drop when insurance companies pay doctors and hospitals the same fee for both natural or c-section deliveries? They do drop—which suggests that a practitioner's economic gain is a significant reason c-sections are often performed.

Some 75 percent of all tranquilizers are prescribed to women. Women are more likely to be on a psychiatrist's couch than are men. Are women by nature more depressed, more mentally deficient, more vulnerable to disease? Of course not!

The fact is that women are the major source of cash flow to American medicine. While there are no exact figures available, estimates say women account for more than $600 billion of the $1 trillion spent annually on health care in America. And it's clear why this is. Women regularly begin seeing a doctor as soon as they reach puberty. Men don't arrive in the waiting room until heart disease occurs or their prostates enlarge. If a man is stressed out or unhappy, he's told to take a vacation. A woman with the same symptoms is told to see a doctor.

And as doctors who treat women are threatened economically by the changes going on in insurance reimbursement, they have found new niches of opportunity to keep their practices lucrative. Cosmetic surgery, of which 90 percent is done on women, is booming. Sports medicine even has a new subspecialty in sports gynecology! Do we need more evidence?

The trail of women as victims of the American medical system is a long one. True, women have been fighting back and are demanding better and safer treatments for real—not imagined—problems. But as long as the medical world— even with the influx of women as doctors—continues to see women's bodies as problems just waiting to be fixed and as big sources of income, treating women as diseases will remain just too good a niche to pass up.

Foxes Guarding the Chicken Coop

Is doctoring an art or a science?

About 10 years ago, I debated this topic with the head of the American Medical Association. We were members of a federal panel trying to come up with ways to assess the quality of individual doctors. The panel included consumer advocates like me, physicians and hospital administrators.

Back then, there was virtually no public information about the competency of individual doctors. Yet there were plenty of stories of incompetent physicians who were jumping from state to state and making headlines in medical malpractice cases.

Still, the AMA chief on the panel argued, it was impossible to come up with standards to compare one doctor to another.

"What do you mean?" I bellowed. "If that's the case, why do states require doctors to pass an examination before awarding them a license to practice? Isn't that a measure of a doctor's ability? And why do medical organizations create boards that certify physician competency in certain specialties? Isn't that sifting out the good from the not-so-good? And on what basis do hospitals choose which doctors are granted privileges? If medicine is strictly an art, then these tests and determinations are hogwash. Why shouldn't consumers know just how well a doctor plies his trade?"

There was a lot of chair squirming going on. "You just don't understand, Charles," he responded. "Unlike with other professionals, it is impossible to compare one doctor with another. In fact, it's something consumers should not worry about!"

Back then, the AMA refused to acknowledge the importance of evaluating doctors. But my, how times have changed. Did you know that this same American Medical Association has now launched a program to accredit doctors, proclaiming that an AMA seal of approval will better protect consumers? It looks at board certification, disciplinary actions, malpractice suits, advanced education and other matters that help determine how competent a doctor really is.

This new initiative is clearly a reaction to pressure, both from consumers and from the managed care industry. You see, ever since that panel broke up—accomplishing nothing, I might add—consumer organizations have been successful in getting federal and state laws passed that are tracking physician and hospital records. These organizations have also been making much of the information public. And most of these laws have been enacted over the strong objection of organized medicine.

Health maintenance organizations are under pressure, too. They must prove to their members that the doctors in their programs really are the best, just like they say in their advertising. As a result, most HMOs have created their own standards for selecting and retaining doctors.

But before you start resting too comfortably in this new consciousness, you should be aware that not very much of the AMA's info will be made public. Instead, the AMA plans to sell the information to managed care companies. That way, HMOs won't need to do as much research to select their doctors. And I'm positive many HMOs will jump at this opportunity because if something goes wrong with one of their contracted doctors, they can blame it on the AMA accreditors.

That's not very reassuring to me. Just a few short years ago, this same group didn't think such information was worth anything. And I'm still not sure it thinks the information is of much value. Remember: The American Medical Association is primarily a trade organization—an entity created to promote its members' interests. This new program is not being done with the public good at heart. Obviously, this is a program to protect doctors. And what are they really protecting doctors from? Customers: whether those customers are consumers or managed care companies.

It remains to be seen just how successful this new program will be. I'm sure it will bring in a lot of cash to the AMA, and the accredited doctors will run around waving their little accreditation certificates. But I'm not so sure the public will buy into this program and accept the AMA seal of approval as a sign of competence. All it will take before all public confidence is eroded are a few headlines showing that an AMA-accredited doctor is committing gross malpractice.

We do need a system that helps consumers choose and use medical practitioners. But that system should not be run by a biased trade association laden with conflicts of interest. It's my view that the federal government should take on the responsibility. What we need is a system that does not just accredit doctors but also certifies their training and competence to do certain procedures. Isn't it time that we require doctors to pass a test of sorts before allowing them to perform coronary bypass surgery, remove a prostate gland or do a hysterectomy? If we start to really look at what a doctor does and how well she does it—and certify her training and competence—we will be providing consumers with not only information but also the reassurance that the people treating them are of the highest quality.

And that's the bottom line, isn't it?

Keeping an Eye Out

Twenty-two years ago, I sat in a federal courtroom in Philadelphia and listened to stories of abuse in nursing homes. Residents testified that nursing home staff routinely burned them with cigarettes, beat them with heavy key chains and neglected to assist them with their personal needs.

Witnesses who had made unannounced visits to these facilities testified that beds often had no sheets or blankets. There was evidence that less-able patients were never bathed. Most residents' possessions were stolen by staff persons. And mentally disabled residents were often shackled to beds and allowed to wallow in their own feces and urine. Rape and other brutalities were common. The situation was pathetic and cried for reform.

In the mid-1970s, these tales of nursing home horror were routine. People placed in long-term care were treated as second-class citizens, with virtually no rights. They were out of sight and, therefore, out of mind.

But slowly, reform began to occur. Advocates for the handicapped and elderly began a concerted effort to force legislators to pass laws that protected the rights of persons in nursing homes. And those efforts have produced significant results. Compared with 20 years ago, long-term care is much improved.

But long-term care is also different than it used to be. The cost of nursing homes, for one, has become exorbitant. One year in a skilled nursing facility, the most medically oriented form of long-term care, can easily cost $70,000 to $100,000. Intermediate care nursing homes, those that provide some medical assistance but primarily serve a person's daily needs, start at $35,000 per year. The vast majority of persons in these two types of long-term care have the bills paid by Medicaid. And that's only after they have already spent most of their assets on their care. In fact, more Medicaid money is spent on formerly middle-class senior citizens living in nursing homes than on ordinary medical care for the poor!

Other long-term-care options are now in place. Home care is available in most areas of the country, with Medicare and Medicaid helping to reimburse the cost if a person is eligible. More affluent persons can move into assisted living communities. These are places that not only provide normal home or apartment living but also have nursing facilities available to assist people who become medically needy. What used to be called retirement centers are beginning to be called congregate living communities. Many of these programs have some medical and living assistance available.

Even with all the reforms and options, most consumers need to be very careful when choosing a facility or program for themselves or a loved one. Abuses exist at every level of long-term care despite government crackdowns. No one really wants to be in long-term care, and no family member ever feels comfortable putting a loved one in such a facility. However, the need for such programs is real. Just as real is the need to be vigilant.

Even with all the rules to protect the rights of patients in long-term care, abuses are happening on a daily basis. You can bet that even as you read this, someone in a nursing home is being hurt by an uncaring or neglectful staff member. That's why it is not only essential that you be careful when you choose a facility but also that you be on patrol after a family member or friend becomes a resident.

The horror stories that unfolded in that courtroom more than two decades ago might never have happened if someone had cared for those people. It's a sad commentary, isn't it, that so many people are left alone at a stage of life that demands so much care and attention.

Who Knows?

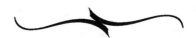

Not long ago, I had a meeting with a vice president for personnel at a large corporation. While waiting to be taken into his office, I struck up a conversation with his secretary. She knew I was involved with health care, so naturally the conversation turned to matters medical. She was telling me just how surprised she was at the number of employees of the corporation who had mental health problems. She told me that in all her years with the company—she had been there more than 25—she had never seen so many people with so many problems.

I asked her how she knew about all these cases since this was a company with many branches in many cities.

"Well," she said, "you know we're self-insured, so all the invoices and reports come through this office."

A few minutes later, I was in her boss's office—a fellow I have known for a long time. I told him of my conversation with his secretary and how surprised I was at her intimate knowledge of the mental health records of the company's employees. Didn't the company have a policy about employee health confidentiality?

He chuckled. "Sure, we have a policy. In fact, nothing is to leave this office. But the problem is, I have 10 people who review all these claims, and human nature being what it is, word will get around."

Word certainly does get around about your medical record. At a meeting I attended in Washington a few years ago, a federal health investigator reported that during a typical hospital stay, 34 of the staff members there will see your medical record. His same report noted that only six needed to see it. More than 20 of these "record Peeping Toms" were billing clerks, file clerks, marketing personnel and other non-medical people.

But the lack of confidentiality about your medical record does not stop there. Every time you get a life insurance physical, the results are sent to the Medical Information Bureau in Massachusetts, which maintains a huge data bank of medical histories. When you apply for a policy, insurance companies go into that data bank to find out your past medical history. Until recently, you wouldn't have known what might be in that record. It wasn't until around 1995 that after much protest, the organization agreed to allow consumers access to their own information. The MIB now also allows you to enter your own side of the story if you disagree with what's in the file.

It seems like everyone has easier access to your medical record than you do. I get 30 to 40 calls a week from people asking about their right to their own records. In most cases, these are people whose doctor or hospital will not give them copies.

So let me set the record straight about your medical history. Twenty-seven states have laws that explicitly give you the right to have copies of your doctor, hospital and mental health records. In the other 23 states, you also have the right to copies of your record. Those states just don't have specific statutes on the books to guarantee it. So no matter where you live, you have the right to a copy of your medical record. Don't let anyone tell you otherwise.

But the key word is "copy." While the record may be about you, the actual record is owned by the health care provider or facility. You are entitled to a copy, not to the original. So, for example, if you want your x-rays, you will be charged for copies to be made. Providers are also allowed to charge reasonable fees for copying other records, as well.

You also have the right to prohibit access to your medical record. You are permitted to inform doctors and hospitals that they are not to release your record to any third party without getting specific permission from you. This includes your employer and insurance companies. You are also entitled to review what is given to anyone else, so you have complete knowledge about what is being released. The point is that you do have control.

Oh, yes, I forgot to tell you something else about that secretary to whom I spoke. After she told me about all of her fellow employees in therapy, I asked if *she* had used any mental health services. She looked at me indignantly and said sternly, "That, Mr. Inlander, is none of your business."

Gag
Orders

"Mr. Inlander!" the doctor roared from the back of the auditorium. "You don't know what you're talking about. Frankly, I'm insulted at your suggestion that I should inform my patients of my record as a physician. I've been practicing medicine for 40 years. My reputation is second to none. Just ask anybody in this room. The fact is that most of my patients are not qualified to determine my competence."

The room began to thunder with applause. There I was, standing before more than 400 doctors, and it was obvious that every one of them was hoping I'd suddenly develop an untreatable terminal illness.

That was Charlotte, North Carolina, on a Saturday morning in the spring of 1988. A medical malpractice insurance company had invited me to speak at a meeting of its local clients. Knowing I would be less of a draw than the golf course, the company promised to give any doctor who attended a 5 percent discount on next year's premium.

After the applause died down, I asked a question of my critical friend.

"What is your specialty?"

"I'm an orthopedic surgeon," he yelled.

Then I turned to the rest of the audience and asked,

"Raise your hand if you hold my friend here in high regard as a surgeon."

Every hand in the room went up.

"Now," I asked, "how many of you have either been his patient or referred someone to him?" Three-quarters of the hands went down.

"Of those with your hands still up," I continued, "how many of you have referred more than two patients to him?" Only three hands remained up. "And of you three, how many of you have asked the patients you referred to him if they were satisfied with the outcome?" Only one hand remained high.

"So," I said, "three hundred and ninety-eight of you think he's a great doctor, but only one of you really knows anything about his track record."

I left the stage to their boos and catcalls.

I was reminded of this entire incident by the controversy over managed care companies imposing so-called gag orders on doctors who work for them. Physicians claimed contractual language prevented them from being able to discuss with their patients the financial restrictions in health maintenance plans that might prohibit doctors from ordering certain tests and services. All across the country, the medical community came together to protest. Some even managed to convince legislators in several states to introduce bills banning gag orders in order to protect the sanctity of the doctor-patient relationship.

Well, all I have to say is this: Doctors may have finally climbed onto the white horse of consumerism, but they're still wearing black hats.

Throughout this century, American doctors have lived under their own self-imposed code of silence. They don't need managed care companies to tape their mouths shut. Think about it: The doctor who *does* fully explain a medical diagnosis, how a prescription works and the details of the procedure he is about to perform is the exception, not the rule. Like the doctor who yelled at me back in 1988, most M.D.'s or D.O.'s don't believe consumers are smart enough to be part of the decision-making process. Not only do doctors keep information away from their patients, they also keep it away from each other. State licensing agency reports consistently show that doctors do not, and will not, turn in colleagues they know are incompetent.

Now that managed care companies have stripped doctors of some of their power, doctors are screaming. But it's all pretty self-serving. What we must do is break all the codes of silence, no matter who imposes them. And while I'm thrilled that doctors are angry about not being allowed to tell consumers about matters important to their treatment or overall health, I wonder just how forthcoming they'd be if they got the power back.

I'd like to go back today and speak to those same doctors in North Carolina. I'm curious to know how they'd respond. Perhaps now they'd like to work with a consumer advocate like me—not because they think I'm entirely right, but because now doctors are starting to realize the importance of talking to more than just themselves.

No Comedy of Errors

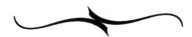

Several years ago, I got into an argument with my family physician and a specialist. The subject was my medical record and an inaccurate test result that I wanted deleted from both doctors' files. Neither doc wanted it out.

Let me explain the situation. Because I was almost 50 at the time, my family physician had suggested I get a prostate-specific antigen blood test, the primary test used to screen for prostate cancer. When the test results came back, my doctor called with a worried voice.

"I think you need to see a urologist," he said. "Your PSA results were in the 12 range, way above the normal level of under four."

I quickly made an appointment with the specialist. He examined me and could find no other symptoms. He suggested a biopsy of the prostate gland. I was hesitant to agree.

"Look," I said, "I think the test result might be in error. Before I have the biopsy, let me get another PSA test, and let's send it to a different lab." The urologist reluctantly agreed.

The new test result came back with a PSA reading under one. And after a few weeks of probing, we discovered that the first lab had mislabeled my blood with the name of an 88-year-old man who had advanced prostate cancer.

That led to my request. Why should erroneous information be kept in my record? Knowing that medical records are viewed by many parties, including insurers and, in some cases, employers, I didn't want false information in my file. But the doctors fought me. They wanted to add a note to the record indicating the first test was wrong. But I stood my ground. And I finally won.

Over the years, I have fielded countless calls and letters from people upset by what is in their medical records—that is, if they could even get copies. One woman could not understand why she was being treated so strangely by doctors for more than a decade. Doing some digging, she found that 10 years earlier, when she had been hospitalized for several days, a doctor had inserted a note in her record describing her as "psychotic." She had questioned her doctor about the need for many of the tests and procedures being performed on her during that stay, and clearly, the doctor had become exasperated with her questions. In fact, she remembered him telling her that she shouldn't act "crazy" about what was happening to her.

Of course, she wasn't crazy or psychotic. She was merely doing what any good medical consumer should be doing—asking questions. But this doc didn't like it. He defined questioning a doctor as being psychotic and wrote it in her record. The problem was that the hospital record was passed along to other doctors. And in time, it was noted in the record of every doctor she saw. No wonder she was treated strangely! It took her years to get these records cleared, and she's still not sure she's taken care of them all.

What most of us don't realize is just how easy it is for a doctor, nurse or almost any other health professional to mislabel us. By merely writing a single word in a medical record, a professional can dramatically affect a patient's life. Imagine the impact of someone indicating that you have a disease you don't have. People have lost their jobs over such incompetence—particularly if that entry deals with an out-of-favor illness or condition.

I'm reminded of my fight because Congress is in the midst of considering ways to guarantee patient privacy in this new era of electronic data transmission. Recommendations are coming from a federal advisory panel that was formed under the Kennedy-Kassebaum health insurance portability law. That's the law that protects workers from losing health insurance simply because they change jobs or because they have a preexisting condition. And it has several provisions addressing the issue of medical privacy. Many other entities, from consumer organizations to health insurers, are also weighing in on the issue.

The issue is significant. Today, most hospitals, doctors and insurers rely upon computer-based medical records to do their jobs. It's very convenient and efficient. When needed, electronic medical information can be shared with medical personnel in minutes practically anywhere around the globe. These records are also easier to read—no notoriously bad handwriting to contend with.

The problem with this medical superhighway, though, is that many more people are now able to view a patient's record—including people who have no medical interest in the case at all. It also means that huge data banks of medical records are rapidly being assembled by managed care companies and other insurers. That, in and of itself, isn't a bad thing, except that there are virtually no state or federal laws regulating how this information can and will be used.

So there is a pressing need for regulation. It must be made crystal clear when, how and why a medical record can be transmitted and who can have access to it. Plus, it is essential that patients be informed in writing who has looked at their files.

Compounding the problem is the difficulty most consumers have gaining access to their medical records. There is no state that prohibits a consumer access to her medical record. In fact, 27 states have actual statutes giving consumers that right. But even in states without declared laws, everyone has a right to a copy of her records.

But doctors and hospitals too often give people a hard time about it. From scowls to $2-per-page copying fees, many doctors and hospitals put up tremendous roadblocks. And some go so far as to give people only a summary of the record, not the complete record itself.

A person's medical record is the health equivalent of a financial credit report. It can make or break a person. In my case, if the erroneous prostate test result had gone off to one of those large life insurance databases, it is likely I would never be able to purchase another life insurance policy in my lifetime. And if another entity inquired of the insurer why I was denied coverage, the error could be catapulted into denied employment.

True, I eventually won the battle to have the error removed from my medical record. But I have no way of knowing if I got to it before cyberspace did. Sometime in the future, this goof could easily come back to haunt me. Frankly, I shouldn't have to put up with that. Nor should anyone else. The last thing in the world we should wonder about when we're sick or in need of medical treatment is if our medical record is wrong.

Step
Right Up

Step right up! Come on, get a little closer. Don't be shy. I've got nothing here that will hurt you. In fact, what this bottle contains will cure your lumbago, ease your tensions and clear your sinuses to boot. And did I mention that this mixture of herbs, directly from the medicinal centers of China, will also shrink those hemorrhoids?

Sounds like an 1890s medicine show, doesn't it? Think of those guys, who usually called themselves Professor Somebody-or-Other, standing on the back of a wagon peddling elixirs loaded with alcohol and a little flavoring. Guaranteed to "fix everything that ails ya," these tonics did little more than empty your pocketbook.

I thought of this when one of the nation's largest health maintenance organizations, Oxford Health Plans, a company that takes in about $3 billion each year, announced that its members in New York, New Jersey and Connecticut would be able to see naturopaths, massage therapists, chiropractors, acupuncturists and other practitioners of complementary medicine. And the company announced plans to sell its own line of over-the-counter herbs and self-care products. Of course, Oxford is the company that made headlines in 1997 when its earnings were far less than anticipated and its stock dropped by half in less than a day. So it remains to be seen just how far this new program will go.

Many insurance companies have started covering certain types of complementary treatment in the past few years, but Oxford is taking it to a new level. And while I like some of what it's doing, such as covering acupuncture and massage therapy, I am not so sure Oxford is acting in best interest of the consumer in other ways.

For example, Oxford subscribers who want to use complementary practitioners have to pay an additional 3 percent on their premium. Why? If these practitioners provide good services at lower prices, it seems Oxford should be offering consumers reduced premiums, not higher ones.

Plus, Oxford says consumers who want to use complementary practitioners don't need to see their primary care practitioner first. Yet the whole idea of the HMO primary care physician is to ensure that patients get the appropriate level of care. Why exempt complementary practitioners and Oxford subscribers from this safeguard? Is it reasonable to expect that a massage therapist will suspect a brain tumor when the patient comes with a headache? I doubt it. Of course, I suspect the real reason Oxford lets consumers bypass the primary care docs is because few allopathic doctors would refer patients to complementary practitioners.

Oxford says *it* selects complementary practitioners, meaning a set of standards are employed to make sure only the best are in the program. I applaud it for that, but I wonder what those standards are. If the standards are like the ones used by most HMOs in selecting doctors, consumers should be wary. The fact is that most HMOs pick doctors by their education, affiliations, lawsuit history and willingness to accept the HMO's payment schedule. Few HMOs know anything about the past clinical competence of the doctors in their program.

And as I noted earlier, Oxford is not in the best of shape. So how much money does it spend to check out the complementary practitioners in its program? I worry that unsuspecting consumers may fall into the hands of poorly trained practitioners or those with less-than-stellar records.

Finally, it bothers me when an insurance company gets into selling medicinal products. Talk about a conflict of interest!

That's why the old medicine show pitch came to mind. It may just be going by a new name.

PART II

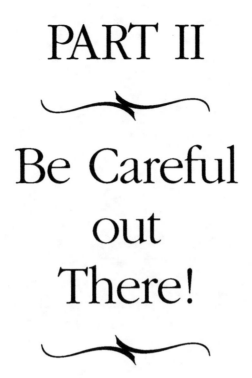

Be Careful out There!

Physicians complain these days about how hard it is to be a doctor. They moan about more paperwork, government regulations, managed care restrictions and skeptical patients. But I'm here to say that being a medical consumer is much more difficult than being a doc. From changes in insurance coverage to conflicting medical opinions about how to treat a medical condition, life for those of us at the other end of the stethoscope is only getting harder.

In this section of the book, I concentrate on getting more from the medical system. Being a savvy medical consumer means having information and being on the lookout for greed and self-interest. This is especially important as we witness a complete change in how health care is delivered through health maintenance organizations and other managed care settings.

Complain, Complain, Complain

I know a man who called the county sheriff when a hospital would not discharge his wife. She had been hospitalized for several days, was fully insured and was told by her doctor she could go home. When she went to the cashier's office to check out, they informed her that she owed less than $50 for incidental expenses not covered by her insurance. She asked to have a bill mailed to her since she had not come to the hospital with a checkbook or cash. The hospital refused to release her until the bill was settled.

Her husband, who was listening to this exchange, went to a nearby pay telephone and called the sheriff's office. He told them his wife was being held for ransom at the local hospital. A few minutes later, a deputy arrived with handcuffs already open. The deputy informed a flustered hospital administrator that ransom was illegal and that unless he discharged the woman, he would be handcuffed and arrested. She was immediately released. And by the way, the next day the hospital changed its policy.

Complaining about shoddy medical care is important.

Nothing will improve unless we consumers speak up. Most people think that doctors and hospitals come under a great deal of scrutiny. Actually, that's far from the truth. Banks are inspected more often than hospitals are. In most states, your car is required to be inspected more often than a hospital's x-ray machines are.

What surprises most people is the fact that doctors are usually never reviewed by government authorities for competence once they've gotten their state licenses! That's right. Once a doctor gets her license, not a single state requires that she ever be examined again. And most states have minimal, if any, continuing education requirements. So it's possible that you have been—or are still being—treated by a doctor who has not only not kept up with her training but may be impaired or incompetent to boot.

That's why complaining is so important. Unless consumers speak up about something that has gone wrong, the chances are that the authorities will never discover it. Several years ago, I was on Oprah Winfrey's show with more than a dozen victims of an obviously less-than-competent doctor. And these women were only a small number of the hundreds he had hurt. How was he able to practice his incompetent trade for years? No one complained. Even other doctors in the town who saw many of the victims after their colleague did his damage did not speak up. As a result, thousands of other women unsuspectingly went to an incompetent doctor. And when something went wrong, the doctor would say that he'd never seen that happen before. It must have been a unique problem associated with that woman. In other words, she was the problem, not him.

Finally, one woman filed a complaint with the state medical licensing board and filed a malpractice suit. The suit was picked up by the media. Within several days, hundreds of other women who had been hurt by the doctor's incompetence came forward. He was later stripped of his license.

If someone had said something earlier, the trail of victims he left might have been shorter. When I spoke to those women on the show, each told me she thought some government organization checked up on doctors on a regular basis.

Most of us have no idea where to turn when we have a complaint about the health care we receive. While every state regulates doctors and hospitals, none makes it easy to file a complaint. Not one state has a toll-free number to lodge a gripe against a hospital. Indiana is the only state that has an 800 number to file charges against a physician.

Here are some tips on where to turn when you are not satisfied with either the quality of the care you receive or the business tactics employed by health care providers.

On matters related to the actual care received, first file a complaint with the appropriate state licensing board. For example, if it's a complaint against a doctor, the complaint should be filed with your state medical licensing board. If it's a hospital complaint, file it with the state hospital licensing board. In addition, most states have licensing or oversight boards dealing with nursing homes, ambulatory care centers and insurance companies (which license health maintenance organizations and other managed care programs). There are also state boards licensing nurses, chiropractors and most other health care practitioners. Get the address at your local library or by calling your state representative. Explain all the details. Provide exact names, dates and the circumstances surrounding the situation. Give the board about two weeks to respond. If you hear nothing, call and ask for an update. If you feel things are not moving, call your state legislator and ask her to intervene. And if you feel you or a loved one has been injured due to negligence or incompetence, don't hesitate to contact a malpractice attorney.

If you have a billing or other business-type problem, contact your local consumer protection agency. Let the Better Business Bureau know about it. Call your state's attorney general if you think fraud or other business laws are being violated.

In addition, your health insurance company may be able to help you with a billing dispute. When you call, ask for the company's fraud division. It will respond faster and with more impact. If you are a Medicare or Medicaid beneficiary, call your U.S. senators or representatives and ask them to look into the matter. Remember: Your congressperson is your Medicare or Medicaid insurance agent.

Health care is a service, and you are entitled to the highest-quality care available. And if something goes wrong, don't be afraid to speak up and speak out.

Negotiate!

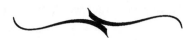

About 10 years ago, my young daughter had an ear infection. We took her to the doctor, who examined her, prescribed an antibiotic and asked us to bring her back in two weeks.

On the way home, fresh from paying close to $40 for less than five minutes' work—this was 10 years ago, remember—I began thinking about that follow-up visit. The doctor would probably peer into her ear for a few seconds, proclaim her infection-free and then charge us another 25 bucks.

By the time we got home, I'd come up with a plan. I phoned the doctor's office and left a message for him to call me when he had some spare time. The next morning, he did.

I told him that I had been thinking about Amy's follow-up visit and that I felt he shouldn't charge us for it unless something was still wrong. In a polite and friendly way, I suggested that the $40 bill from the day before should cover the next visit, as well. Then I held my breath, ready for a major argument. In fact, I'd already begun thinking of other doctors we might turn to if we couldn't work something out with this one.

Much to my surprise, the doctor agreed to my terms. In fact, he told me that he thought my request was reasonable. He said that our business was very important to him and that he did not want to lose it. Since then, I have negotiated often with doctors.

As our health care system changes, so must our thinking about how we interact with it. Medicine has become big business, and we are the customers. Today, more than 80 percent of all physicians are either employees of a managed care company or are under contract with one. So, for better or worse, when we visit a doctor, we are also visiting a corporation. And negotiating with a corporation or a business is pretty routine.

Negotiating does not mean fighting. It means working out an arrangement that is agreeable and comfortable for both sides. Negotiating is a method of developing a partnership with another party. And the basis of any doctor-consumer relationship should be a partnership.

Negotiating also produces other benefits. When both sides feel comfortable with each other, particularly when each agrees with what is going to happen, there is a greater sense of respect for one another. And respect in the doctor-consumer relationship is essential. But that respect should not be one-way, meaning it should not just be the consumer respecting the doctor. A sound relationship is one in which there is mutual respect. The physician should respect the consumer's wishes and beliefs and not simply expect reverence and deference from others.

Another benefit is one's own sense of control. As consumers, we often grant control to a health care professional without thinking. That makes us more vulnerable to having our wishes overlooked. Negotiating with a health care provider ensures that the relationship is the partnership it should be—while still maintaining each side's personal integrity.

For many years, I've been recommending that consumers negotiate with their doctors. And for many years, I've been getting positive feedback from people who do it.

Back in the 1970s, I was involved with moving citizens who were mentally retarded from large, warehouselike public institutions into more habilitating, community-based group homes. At one of the institutions, a place with more than 1,000 residents, one woman was discovered to have breast cancer. Upon further examination, it was found that the cancer had spread to her lymph nodes. This woman was in her late 60s and had been a resident of the institution for more than 50 years. Not only did she not want to leave the facility, but she also did not want to go through the operation. She was afraid of the operation and sensed that the quality of her life after surgery was not going to be very good, either. And despite her inability to read and her very deliberate way of communicating, she tried to tell the doctor that she would rather die than go through that misery.

The institution doctor would hear nothing of it. She was not bright enough to make such a decision. This was a medical problem! How could a person with a low IQ—one who had been institutionalized for the vast majority of her life— make an informed decision?

I was called in on the situation. I immediately asked the court, which was overseeing the movement of the residents to the community, to hold a hearing on the matter. The woman, the doctor, several lawyers and I were present with the judge a few days later. The judge asked the doctor to describe the situation. He explained the woman's condition and why surgery gave her the best hope. He explained that unless she had the surgery, she would probably die within six months. With the surgery, he could not be sure.

The judge asked the woman to come forward. He asked her if she understood what was happening. She said yes. She said that if she didn't have this operation, she would probably die. And if she did have the operation, she might live a little longer, but she would not be able to do many of the things she liked to do. She said she would rather die than be in that state.

The judge then asked her about her conversations with the doctor. She said that the doctor never really listened to her. He kept insisting she have the surgery. When she asked him if there was anything else he could do, he would bark a loud NO!

The judge took a short recess and came back. He told the doctor that the woman had every right to make the decision she did and that she fully understood the consequences of her actions.

"But," he added quite sternly to the doctor, "you failed to give her options. You failed to negotiate what could be done for her despite her decision."

The judge rebuked the doctor for not telling the woman what options she had if the pain got worse. He told the doctor that his role was not to dictate, but to negotiate.

Seven months later, the woman died. But in the interim, she and the doctor had built a strong and close relationship. When she was having problems, he would describe what could be done. Together they made decisions. When he felt strongly about a certain course of care, he would make his case, but oftentimes, she said no or opted for something else.

After she died, I had a meeting with the doctor on another matter. As I was leaving, I asked him how he felt about what had happened over the past months. He surprised me with his answer. He said that the judge had awakened him to a major shortcoming in his dealings with patients. He had never thought about medical care being the outcome of a negotiation, but that upon reflection, he realized that it was the best way to go.

I couldn't agree more.

Cold Sweat

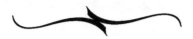

I had a horrible nightmare. I woke up in a cold sweat, my teeth clenched and every muscle in near spasm. I threw off the covers and stared quietly at the ceiling until I calmed down. I've had bad dreams before, but this was clearly the worst.

The dream started benignly enough. I was shopping for a new suit at a major department store. I found one that I liked and took it back to the fitting room to try it on. It looked great on me, so I decided to buy it. The salesperson brought out the tailor to mark the suit up for alterations.

The tailor was a nice-looking, older gentleman who wore a white smock with large pockets. He took out his marking chalk and a few pins and started with the jacket. He then moved to the slacks. He marked them at the waist, then for length. I thought he was done, so I started to get down from his little podium. But he stopped me.

"Wait a minute, mister!" he said. "We have a special going on right now."

He proceeded to pull a pair of latex gloves out of his pockets and put them on.

"For every suit purchased this week, the store is offering a free digital exam for prostate enlargement. So just bend over, and we'll check it out."

That's when I woke up.

Now I'm no Freud, but I know exactly what prompted that dream. That day I had received a press release from two suburban Chicago hospitals announcing the opening of a mammography center at a Nordstrom's department store. It was the first such facility of its kind ever to open in a retail store. The center opened in October 1995—October is breast cancer awareness month—and guess what? If you came in for a mammogram before October 31, you got a special discount. They also offered four free breast health seminars. I'm sure they took most insurance, and I'll bet credit cards were graciously accepted.

Frankly, the idea of bringing medical testing and screening to the consumer is a good idea, and it's not entirely new. About 20 years ago, we began seeing blood pressure machines in malls. For a quarter, you could get your blood pressure checked, and one study found that some mall machines were more accurate than tests done by doctors.

Not all medical testing in malls or stores is reliable. Cholesterol screenings—usually sponsored by hospitals—have been criticized for taking blood samples in invalid and sometimes unsanitary ways.

But overall, the movement to bring medical testing out of the laboratory and into stores and public places has been helpful and healthful. More people get tested and screened for conditions today than ever before. And having these services available in public places, such as malls, raises awareness about the importance of prevention.

If there is a downside to all this, it may only be an increase in the medical paranoia that exists in America. Sure, we want to detect breast cancer early—catching any major medical problem sooner rather than later can improve a person's chance of fighting and beating a disease. But I'd hate to see medicine spill over into every corner of life. Occasionally, all of us just need a break. So while I'm glad that consumers can buy a hat and then get a mammogram at Nordstrom's—it may be a while before many women consider that a treat.

How Qualified Is Your Doctor?

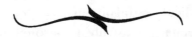

Not long ago, I received a letter from an angry woman. For more than a year, she had been attending therapy sessions with a psychiatrist to help her overcome the loss of a child. She had lapsed into deep depression after her son's death and had sought professional help. The psychiatrist she was using came highly recommended by her family doctor. She had been told the psychiatrist specialized in individual therapy and had a large clientele from the local area.

She began her sessions almost immediately after being referred. She liked the doctor, but after four or five months, she was concerned by her lack of progress. Her sessions were not going anywhere, and the medication he had prescribed for her seemed to have little effect.

When she confronted the psychiatrist about this, he told her to be patient. "It takes time," he said.

She continued under his guidance, but when a full year

had passed and her depression and feelings of sadness had not subsided, she decided to seek a change. She called the local mental health association and asked for a listing of physicians and other therapists in the area who might be of assistance. When she received the list, she was surprised to find that her current psychiatrist was not listed. She called to ask why he was not on the list and was informed that while he was indeed a licensed physician, he did not have enough psychiatric training to warrant the organization's recommendation.

She was startled! "But he's a psychiatrist," she said. "How could he not have enough training?"

And she was more startled by the response. "Oh," she was informed, "any physician can call himself anything he wants. This doctor happens to call himself a psychiatrist."

Maybe you're surprised, as well. But the fact is that once a physician receives a medical license, he can call himself anything. From surgeon to psychiatrist, no state puts any restrictions on what a licensed physician may claim as a specialty. In fact, in some cases, doctors have been known to make up specialties out of thin air.

Does that mean that all doctors claim specialties without having gone through the training? No. In fact, most doctors have received advanced training in one or more areas. But it's important that you check out your doctor's credentials and training before you agree to be a patient.

Here are some things to look for. First, find out if the doctor is board certified in her specialty. Board certification means the doctor has taken advanced training, has passed additional examinations and regularly attends continuing education. It does not guarantee competence, but it does demonstrate a higher level of commitment to the specialty.

Next, find out where the doctor has hospital privileges. Then, call the hospital and ask in what area of specialty the doctor works. This is a good way to verify a physician's claim because hospitals usually will not grant privileges to doctors without the necessary advanced training.

Find out about your doctor's education. From where she went to medical school to the internships and residencies she had, ask the doctor about her training and history. And if you are in doubt, call those institutions to check it out.

Check with your state's medical licensing board. See if it has taken any action against the doctor. These boards are usually located in your state capital.

If you're wondering if doing these things makes a difference, consider this. The lady who wrote me checked out her first psychiatrist after the fact. She found out he was not board certified, had no privileges at any hospital, had done no psychiatric residency and had several complaints filed against him at the state level.

And I'm pleased to report that after only a month with a new practitioner, one whom she thoroughly checked out in advance, she was doing fine and later made a full recovery.

Making Sense out of Medical Research

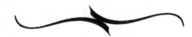

When I was growing up, my father and I had eggs every morning for breakfast. The whole family put sugar on the breakfast cereal. For lunch, we ate hamburgers or cheese sandwiches. We had meat and potatoes and vegetables every night for dinner. On Sundays, we would bring in Chinese food so that my mother would have a break from cooking. A great treat was going to an Italian restaurant for spaghetti and meatballs.

To my mother, this was healthy eating—hearty meals that conformed to doctors' advice and the latest health information reported in newspapers or magazines.

She used to tell me the value of good nutrition, pointing out that with the diet we ate, we would live longer.

I followed my mother's advice for years. But after I graduated from college in the late 1960s, I started paying attention to what the nation's most esteemed medical researchers had to say about diet. Based on what I heard, I stopped eating eggs for breakfast. I stopped adding sugar to everything. And when my daughter was born, we kept her away from sweets, partially to avoid hyperactivity. Red meat became taboo, as did chicken skin, whole milk and other products that would raise cholesterol. Even Chinese and Italian food became less appealing as reports began to surface that many of my favorite dishes were laden with fat.

Yet even while I tried to eat right or better, I kept wondering why my parents and their friends were living well into their 80s given the diets they'd followed for so many years. And why had my grandparents, all of whom survived into their mid-70s and 80s, lived so long on their questionable diets?

So I confess that over the past 10 years, I've developed a healthy skepticism about nutritional advice, in part due to all the conflicting findings. In the last decade, for example, coffee has gone from the good list to the bad list, back to the good list and on to the "we're not sure" list. Scientists also aren't so sure anymore whether high cholesterol causes the increased risk for heart disease they previously believed it did, or whether cutting down on salt is as beneficial for people with high blood pressure as was previously thought.

And then in November 1995, there were two new studies on nutrition that turned previous studies on their heads. The first said, in effect, that eggs aren't a dangerous source of cholesterol after all. Yessiree, even if you have a cholesterol level as high as 250 mg/dl, two eggs a day won't hurt you! The second report suggested that sugar has nothing to do with hyperactivity in children. In other words, when the kids are flying off the walls after coming home from trick-or-treating, it's the excitement of scaring old Mrs. Maloney down the street—not the chocolate—that's to blame.

I have learned several lessons from all of this that I think are beneficial. First, one or even several medical studies are not necessarily the last word on a subject. Second, it's going to take a large body of evidence, looked at over many years, before anyone can claim anything definitive about the relationship between nutrition and disease. And last but not least, I've learned that as usual, my mother has probably had it right all along.

Choosing
Managed
Care

Managed care is getting mixed reviews from consumers, according to a 1996 survey of Chicago area employees. In the survey, 84 percent said they were satisfied with their health maintenance organizations. However, the survey also reported that employees were less satisfied with the programs that required greater out-of-pocket expenses. And another survey of managed care customers conducted by the Commonwealth Fund found a significant percentage were dissatisfied with managed care. Those employees who were forced into a program were especially dissatisfied.

Still, managed care is here to stay and growing. Employers like it because it saves them money. The federal government likes the cost savings and is encouraging Medicare and Medicaid beneficiaries to join approved health maintenance organizations. Up until 1997, health insurance companies loved managed care because it yielded incredible profits. But that's changing, and with those changes will come others in the managed care landscape.

What's happened to cause managed care profits to "go

south"? The number one reason is that managed care companies are now having to treat sick people. Sounds obvious, doesn't it? But most managed care companies are so new that up until recently, they had very few sick people enrolled in their programs. In fact, managed care companies went out of their way looking for enrollees who were younger and less likely to be in need of costly medical services. One managed care executive told me that his company avoided sending sales materials or agents to companies with older populations. And many managed care firms avoided small businesses, especially of the Mom-and-Pop variety, because they tended to have older, usually sicker employees.

Plus, managed care companies were also benefiting from the discounts they were able to get from hospitals and physicians. The discounts came as managed care firms promised facilities and practitioners a high volume of customers in return for lower fees. As a result, HMOs and other managed care plans were saving money long before they passed those discounts on to their customers in the form of lower premiums. It's similar to the "spread" banks use, in which they take your money and get to use it a few days before you have full access to it. The difference between money spent on medical care and the amount collected in premiums created big profits.

But by 1997, managed care had become commonplace. Almost 70 percent of the population was in some form of managed care plan. More than 55 percent were in HMOs alone. That meant that the easy days were over. Fewer new people were joining managed care plans since most were already enrolled. And with the large number of enrollees, it was just a matter of time before they started using the medical services for costly care. Plus, the discounts had already been gotten. There were no more to be had. So managed care companies began losing profits because they had to pay for care at a higher rate and were unable to raise premiums or attract a large number of new enrollees.

The implications of this major change are many—especially for the health care consumer. Aside from worry about what will inevitably be an increase in premiums, there has to be worry about cuts in services or reductions in quality. It is highly likely that some of the services many HMOs offer now will be cut back or eliminated completely in years to come. Or managed care plans may ask consumers to pay an extra premium if they want certain services such as vision care or access to alternative practitioners. And even more worrisome is the possibility that as economic pressures build on managed care plans, they will coerce practitioners and facilities to do less or cut corners in patient care. And that will clearly jeopardize quality.

For most consumers, the major issue is quality. And it is quality that every consumer should look for and monitor when choosing or using a managed care plan.

So what can you do to improve your chances of choosing a managed care program that will deliver the highest quality of care?

First, make sure you choose a program that has been operating for at least three years. Brand-new HMOs and preferred provider organizations have a history of problems with quality. They often have a small network of doctors, a limited number of hospitals and few arrangements for care if you need medical attention away from home.

Choose a plan that has a large number of doctors in it. The more primary care physicians in the program, the greater your choice. The primary care doctor is still the centerpiece of a managed care program. That's because most people's medical needs can be handled by a competent primary care practitioner and because, in most cases, he gives you access to a plan's listed specialists. A good managed care program should have at least three specialists to choose from in any given field. The last thing in the world you want is to be stuck with a specialist you do not like or whose medical judgement you question.

Make sure the program you choose permits you to go outside the network. This is especially important if you travel or need medical services that aren't available close to home. For example, national managed care companies such as Prudential or Kaiser tend to offer more extensive services than do companies that are locally owned and operated.

Don't assume *any* managed care company has chosen the best doctors and hospitals in town. The fact is that most companies contract with any doctor or hospital willing to accept their payment terms. So check out the list of doctors who participate in the program, and ask the managed care company to provide a summary of each doctor's qualifications.

Also, be wary of so-called report cards issued by managed care companies. Most of these report cards tell you very little about the quality of the program's practitioners and facilities.

Finally, before you choose a managed care program, call your state's insurance department, the Better Business Bureau and your state's consumer protection agency to see if there have been complaints filed against the managed care company.

There are many different managed care models to choose from, from HMOs to the newer point-of-service plans, and the quality from one company to another varies greatly. So it's important to know everything possible about the programs that are available to you.

Do Like
My Mother

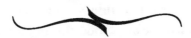

My mother, who is in her late 80s, doesn't like it when a young doctor calls her by her first name. She says it's a sign of disrespect. She feels that someone half her age, whom she has hired to provide medical services, should only use her first name if she invites him to do so. And if you know my mother, you also know that the medical culprit who unwittingly calls her Betty on their first encounter will never do it again.

Unlike most of us, my mother is not intimidated by doctors and other medical professionals. To her, the initials M.D. or D.O. after a name are a sign of training, not ordination. She tends to ignore all the things doctors and hospitals do to make us feel like less-than-worthy participants in our own health care. And given the fact that she's hearty and healthy at her age, she must be doing something right.

It is difficult to overcome the intimidation many of us face when dealing with the world of medicine. Doctors speak in a language most of us don't understand. Instead of just calling it a heart attack, like the rest of us do, doctors label it a "myocardial infarction." I've seen dermatologists running around with stethoscopes sticking out of their pockets. Frankly, I didn't know that pimples made noise. And I have always wondered why psychiatrists wear white coats. What's going to spill on their $800 suits other than some gourmet coffee? A physician calling us by our first name while expecting to be addressed as "doctor" is just as intimidating.

A routine visit to a doctor's office is intimidating, too. Most of us don't see the doctor until after we have taken our clothes off and have sat restlessly on a cold examining table for what seems like hours. Once the doctor arrives, we are more concerned about covering our vital parts than we are about having a meaningful medical discussion. And even if we overcome our modesty, we get very little "talk" time. Studies show that physicians interrupt their patients an average of 18 seconds after they ask what is wrong.

A good doctor-patient relationship is based on mutual respect. One side should not hold all the cards. But if you want things to change, it will be up to you.

Here are some quick ideas to help lower your susceptibility to medical intimidation. Next time you visit the doctor, don't get undressed until after he has come into the room. Make a list of questions, and tell the doctor you expect to have them answered before you leave. Let the doctor know that while you respect him, you'd feel more comfortable with an independent second opinion before you proceed with any major or invasive treatments. If you're bothered by your doctor and his staff calling you by your first name, ask them to call you Mr., Mrs., Ms. or whatever you like. Such a request may serve as a wake-up call to their informality. And finally, take a family member or friend into the examining room with you. This is especially important if you are sick or worried and are not up to asking questions or taking in everything the doctor might tell you.

Do these tactics work? You bet they do. My mother has tried every one of them.

Hospital Rankings

About a year ago, a friend invited me and several others to join him for dinner at one of New York City's most famous restaurants. It has been ranked as one of the top five eateries in the nation for at least 15 years. I graciously accepted the invitation.

When we arrived at the restaurant, we were informed that our table was not ready. "Just a slight delay," the maître d' told us. Forty-five minutes later, we were still waiting. My friend had to make a scene to finally get us seated.

That didn't end the problems. We were informed by the waiter that three items on the menu were no longer available. But it was only 7:30, early by New York dining standards. And what we did order turned out to be awful. Each of us had a different entrée, and no one was satisfied. Two of our party sent their plates back. All in all, it was a miserable meal that cost my host $400 for five people. And when I left that night, I was longing for a great turkey sandwich from that little, inexpensive deli not far from my home in Pennsylvania.

Later, I asked myself how a restaurant like that could be ranked as one of the best. Was the reviewer related to the chef? Did we hit a bad night? Were our tastes too pedestrian?

I am always reminded of this saga when I see the book

from the editors of *U.S. News and World Report.* It's called *America's Best Hospitals,* and it ranks more than 1,000 facilities, covering all 50 states and 10 metropolitan areas. It's an expansion of the magazine's annual *Best Hospitals* guide.

There is much I like about the book. It's especially useful if you're looking for the name of a hospital known for treating certain diseases, such as cancer or heart disease.

But do these rankings mean that you will have a better outcome if you choose a higher-rated facility over a lower-rated one? And what if you choose a hospital that isn't even rated— perhaps one of the 4,000 facilities not reviewed in the publication? Will your chances of a successful result be even lower?

The answer to both questions is no. In fact, even some of the highest-rated facilities have had their share of problems. For example, I discovered that two of the three hospitals that rated highest in the cancer category had made headlines in recent years for major goof-ups. One caused the death of a patient by giving her a massive overdose of medication. The other institution hit the front page when one of its physicians accidentally operated on the wrong side of a woman's brain. And these were not the only highly ranked hospitals in which serious mistakes occurred.

As to the unrated hospitals, the irony is that they may be better for you than some of the greatly touted medical centers. That's because most hospitals these days, big or small, are pretty similar. They've all got the latest advanced technology, allowing them to perform procedures that have become fairly routine. You don't need to go to the Mayo Clinic, for example, to have your gallbladder removed. Nor do you need to be exposed to greater rates of infections or be subject to the poking and probing of medical students so often found in the big university medical centers. In other words, you don't necessarily need the big reputation medical center for most routine, common problems. And in fact, you may find a well-equipped community hospital quieter, more concerned about you and possibly even less of a risk for infection or medical mistake.

View hospital ratings as another bit of information to consider before you make a medical decision. If your problem is unique or complicated, one of these facilities may be the place to turn for either information or treatment. But remember that hospital ratings are *not* based on a review of patient records, just as most restaurant ratings are *not* based on a poll of diners.

And speaking of food again, whether you're dining out or entering the hospital, it's probably a good idea to bring your own turkey sandwich.

The War
for Patients

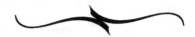

I got a call from a friend of my mother not long ago. For many years, she's had a heart condition, during which time she's used the same cardiologist. When she last visited him, he asked her if she was still seeing her primary care doctor. When she told him yes, the cardiologist suggested she give up the primary doctor. He told her he could take care of most of her problems, and if she needed other specialty care, she could turn to his network of medical colleagues.

As much as she liked the cardiologist and felt good about his care, she was skeptical.

"Why," she asked, "would I want to do that? I'm quite satisfied with my primary care doctor."

"Well," he replied, "coming to me for your primary needs would make your life easier—you wouldn't have to make extra trips to other doctors, and I could better monitor how your overall health might be affecting your heart."

My mother's friend said she would consider it and then called me.

I've heard from many consumers about similar propositions from specialists. In fact, it seems to be a growing trend. I've dubbed it "the war for patients" because, for the first time in our history, we have an enormous glut of doctors, most of them specialists. That means there are too many doctors trying to serve too few patients. In fact, federal studies of physician manpower done each year suggest that as of 1997, 200,000 of the nation's 600,000 physicians are unnecessary.

The government has also taken some action to try to decrease this physician oversupply. In late 1997, the federal government announced that it would pay teaching hospitals to train fewer residents. The logic here was that part of the excess comes from hospitals trying to fill their physician residency programs, which are often funded by the federal government. Now, by paying hospitals to not train a portion of those positions, the government hopes to help the surplus correct itself. It remains to be seen if this will work.

In the meantime, consumers still are faced with too many practitioners. And what that means is that many doctors will do whatever they can to keep their practices lucrative and growing. And that's what the war for patients is all about.

This war for the patient takes many forms. One woman told me about an ophthalmologist who recommended certain vitamins for her macular degeneration that could only be bought from him. That turned out not to be true. The same vitamins were available at a drugstore for a lot less money. The woman was convinced that the doctor was trying to make her ultradependent on his care. It didn't work.

Also, ob-gyns are now fighting with managed care companies to be classified as primary care doctors. They're also worried about retaining patients.

But competition among physicians is not the only thing worrying doctors. They also fear nurses. Advanced practice nurses—professionals such as nurse practitioners—are moving into primary care. Every state allows nurse practitioners to set up independent practices, and although some states do require these highly skilled nurses to work with an agreement with a physician, most states do not invoke this restriction. All states with the exception of Illinois allow advanced practice nurses to write certain types of prescriptions. In other words, it is not just one type of doctor who now threatens to draw patients away from another: Nurses are now in the game, too.

And managed care plans are contributing to the situation. Throughout the country, managed care plans are contracting directly with independent nurse practitioners, asking them to serve as the primary care gatekeepers. They also restrict patient choice, which puts a damper on competition from specialists. Most managed care plans shun the idea that a specialist treat any condition outside his specialty. So if my mother's friend were in a health maintenance organization, it's likely her plan would not allow her to see her cardiologist if she needed treatment for the flu or a minor infection.

Obviously, consumers are caught on the horns of this dilemma. While the specialists, primary care doctors and nurses battle it out, we become the pawns. What may sound like a specialist's concern for our physical well-being may, in fact, be nothing more than a physician's personal concern for his own financial well-being. In today's medical world, practitioner survival has become as important as patient care.

So how do we protect ourselves while they battle it out? The next time your specialist pops the question—can I be your primary care doc?—my advice is to say no. Primary care physicians, whether internists, family or general practitioners, are better trained and more experienced in identifying and treating a wider range of medical problems than specialists are. Plus, they charge less. And nurse practitioners are considered by many medical experts to be as qualified for most primary care needs as doctors in the field.

Second, only use specialists when the problem is clearly in their area of expertise. The more specialized a physician is, the less likely it is she will know about other illnesses and treatments.

Third, don't be pressured to make a change. The doctor glut has turned many good doctors into marketers, and often they cross the ethical line out of fear of losing business.

By the way, my mother's friend said no to her cardiologist and told him that she would stop coming to him before she would give up her primary care doctor.

Listen Up

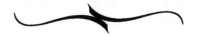

"Well, here's what happened, doctor.

"Last night, I woke up at about three in the morning. I had this pain in my stomach. It was bad. I thought it must have been something I ate for dinner. I went to the bathroom to look for an antacid in the medicine cabinet. The pain was getting worse and I was ..."

What you've just read would take about 18 seconds to say out loud. Now use your imagination and pretend that I've been the typical medical consumer describing a health problem to my doctor. Why did I stop after just 18 seconds? Well, that's typical, too. Several studies on the subject, done over the past two decades, show that on average, consumers have that generous amount of time to tell a doctor what's wrong before the doctor interrupts. And it's downhill from there—patients usually don't get the opportunity to speak again.

Over the years, more people complain to me about this failed communication than anything else. Consumers feel slighted by their physicians and guilty for talking or asking questions.

One recourse consumers seek to this problem is to sue if *anything* goes wrong with their treatment. Yet those doctors who have been sued don't seem to get the message or get any better. One recent study, reported in 1997, found that primary care doctors who had past claims against them spent less time with patients than those who had never been sued. And the sued doctors were less likely to explain what the patient could expect in the course of treatment. These doctors also asked fewer questions and did little to develop a friendly rapport with the patient.

What's particularly worrisome about all this is that current trends in medicine may make this problem even worse and make it next to impossible for doctors who value communicating with patients to do so. Many managed care companies now ask doctors to see a certain number of patients per hour. Doctors complain that if they spend more than 15 minutes with a patient, they are penalized by the health maintenance organization—because HMOs often tie hourly quotas to end-of-the-year bonuses in order to increase efficiency.

Managed care companies, using the old bromide from the 1980s, claim it's the "quality time" spent with a patient, not the quantity, that's important. And they throw the time patients spend with nurses and physician assistants into the "quality time" stew. Yet as important as these other encounters are, nurses and physician assistants often cannot legally determine a patient's course of treatment. And most are instructed not to discuss treatment options or outcomes with patients.

Now don't jump to the conclusion that if we would just do away with managed care, the doctor-consumer communication problems would go away. Sorry, that's just wishful thinking. The "18 seconds" studies were all done in non-HMO settings. The point is simply that doctors are not good listeners.

Most doctors will say that they are good listeners. The problem, according to many physicians, is that patients are not good "tellers." Doctors tell me that most of their customers are not very precise in relating their problems. Consumers tend to hem and haw, giving vague descriptions. That's why they interrupt. They're trying to pinpoint what's wrong without wasting time.

Well, I'm sure there's some truth to their argument, but I'm still not convinced. I've heard from too many consumers, too many times, how they could hardly get their first words out before the doctor barged in with either a diagnosis or a question. And often, these interruptions lead to the patient forgetting to tell the doctor something that was important.

One of the side effects this behavior engenders is a reluctance on the part of many people to be honest or forthright with their doctors. People become intimidated by someone who interrupts—especially someone as authoritative as a physician. As a result, folks become fearful of coming across as stupid or frivolous.

The problem is that we're not going to change doctors by having HMOs change their policies or by offering better courses in medical school. No—the way to change their behavior is to change ours. If we change our tactics, they'll change theirs. They'll have to—we're the only customers they've got.

So here's how to get the attention *and* information you need.

The best thing to do is make a list of the important things you want to tell your doctor and the questions you want answered. Take the list with you to your appointment, and tell the doctor you have a series of points and questions you want to go over. Don't let the doctor leave until you're satisfied and have had your questions answered. Studies show that the better prepared you are for your appointment, the more likely you are to get the attention and information you need. If the doctor gives you a hard time about your list of questions, let him know that there are other doctors out there. And don't be afraid to consider switching doctors if you are not getting the attention and answers you're looking for.

There have been studies that suggest that patients who ask the most questions tend to get the best care. So do not be intimidated by how rushed or important the doctor seems to be. But on the other hand, don't waste the doctor's time, either. Try to make your questions and explanations as brief and precise as possible. And if you have some questions that do not need immediate answers, give them to the doctor in writing and ask him to call you when it's convenient to discuss them.

For most consumers, this is a new way to approach physicians. Don't be afraid to try it. From all the reports I see, it works far more often than not.

It's ironic that all the changes going on in health care are supposed to be making life better for the medical consumer. Yet the practice of the most basic and important part of the doctor-patient relationship—communication—may actually be getting worse. Don't let it happen to you.

Better Than Bearable

I got a very depressing letter from my parents. They're in their late 80s and live independently in Florida. They had just returned from visiting a friend, a widower who had moved into an assisted living community because he was losing his short-term memory and getting confused. Assisted living communities offer residents normal home or apartment living, but they also provide medical services for people with special needs. The particular facility my parents' friend lives in has a great reputation.

Which is why my mother was so shocked by what she saw. In her letter describing the visit, she writes this:

"The place was God-awful. Each patient has a *cell* big enough for a single bed and a chair and a small table and a television. I was really shocked. Everyone is in a wheelchair. He was the only person I saw who was ambulatory. He really is in the wrong place. He's not too confused and can carry on a conversation with good sense. Because he lived alone, he probably could use assisted care, but where he is now reminds me of the movie *One Flew Over the Cuckoo's Nest.*

If he wasn't bad when he went in, he'll certainly end up in bad shape."

Over the years, I have received hundreds of letters similar to this one from my mother. People hate nursing homes. We are repulsed by the thought of losing our dignity, living with others in a frail condition, waiting to die. After a lifetime of hard work and sacrifice, most folks would rather visit Dr. Kevorkian than be placed in some sterile nursing residence.

But nursing homes and other long-term-care facilities are not going to disappear. As much as we hate them, we need them. With both spouses working and families scattered all across the country, we are increasingly unable to take care of our own.

Until Medicare and Medicaid came along, paying for nursing home care was the biggest worry. But with those two programs and private long-term-care insurance, costs, while high, are less of a barrier. What most people worry about is quality. They fear being left to wallow in a warehouse of human suffering. That's clearly what my mother felt when she visited her friend.

Still, compared with 20 years ago, long-term care has improved dramatically. In the 1970s and 1980s, newspapers were filled with horror stories of nursing home residents abused and neglected by uncaring and undertrained staff. Reforms quickly followed. Today, facility staff tend to be better trained, and oversight is more frequent. But we all still need to be vigilant.

Here are some tips you can use to help make the right long-term-care decision. First, with the government putting new restrictions on shifting assets to other family members, consider buying long-term-care insurance. These policies are vastly improved compared with those of a decade ago. The younger you are when you buy one, the cheaper it will be. Such policies are a legitimate way to protect your assets and assure coverage.

If you or a loved one needs home care, only use agencies that are fully accredited. Accredited agencies meet the highest standards in the industry. When choosing a nursing home, pick one where family and friends can visit regularly. Even with all the rules and regulations now in place, abuse and neglect happen. But they are less likely to happen to residents who are visited regularly by people who care.

Also be sure to check out any program or community personally. Don't believe brochures or salespeople. Remember: Most long-term care is provided by profit-making companies that must balance resident care and shareholder returns. Too often, the shareholders become the top priority. But also do not be lulled into complacency by facilities operated by non-profit organizations, including church-related groups. They are just as likely to be neglectful as profit-making programs. Be watchful and wary, no matter how good the place looks.

Also look for telltale signs of neglect when you visit a facility. Are residents tied into their wheelchairs? Many places tie people into wheelchairs not because they might fall out, but rather because they want to make sure that they do not get up and walk around. That's done for the convenience of the staff, not for the benefit of the resident.

If the person being placed into a facility is mentally incapacitated, possibly with Alzheimer's disease or another form of dementia, be extra careful about where she is placed. Just because a home operates a so-called Alzheimer's unit, it doesn't mean that you don't have to really watch what is done there. Oftentimes, such a unit is operated as a human warehouse providing little stimulation to the consumer. Be sure to see what programs are provided, and check out those programs with some surprise visits.

I once visited an elderly woman living in a nursing home operated by a religious order. It was a beautiful sunny day, but she had the curtains drawn tightly across her window.

"It's lovely out," I said. "Why don't you open your curtains and let the sun shine in?"

She smiled slightly and pulled the curtains open. In the distance, you could see a church, and in the foreground was the church cemetery.

"I'll tell you, Charlie," she said pointing at the cemetery. "I can't bear looking out at my next home."

This is a tough stage for all elderly Americans. But it can and should be better than bearable.

Win-Win

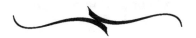

An angry physician criticized me recently for recommending that medical consumers negotiate fees—and even medical treatments—with their doctors. You see, it is my contention that no matter how you look at it, American medicine is a business. And because it is a business, we on the other end of the stethoscope have every right to deal with doctors and medical facilities in a businesslike way. I'm convinced that if the majority of consumers negotiated with their practitioners, the costs of health care would be lower and the quality higher.

I see nothing wrong with negotiating with my doctor. In fact, the art of negotiating is designed to bring parties to the best solution to a problem. And finding the best solution to a personal health care problem couldn't be more critical.

Why is negotiating with your doctor important? In today's high-tech medical world, there are often a variety of ways to deal with a particular medical condition. For some conditions, such as gallstones, there are several surgical and nonsurgical treatment options available. Yet studies show that physicians are not always giving their patients the full range of options from which to choose.

Negotiating also tends to protect a person from unnecessary procedures. Experts estimate that up to a third of all coronary bypass operations are unnecessary, that at least three out of every five cesarean sections are unwarranted and that possibly nine out of 10 hysterectomies should not be performed. If consumers sit down and negotiate the various options with their doctors at the time a procedure is rec-

---

ommended, the likelihood of unnecessary treatment being performed dwindles.

Negotiation is built upon openness. Each side comes to the problem with a different amount of information and a different reason for being there. But both parties want to come to the best resolution. By negotiating medical treatment and care, doctors and consumers have more information to deal with and, in turn, can make decisions that are the most appropriate given the situation.

The same holds true about fee negotiation. Doctors' fees are not written in stone. In fact, most doctors accept different amounts of payment for the very same procedure, depending on who is paying. If Medicare and private insurers are negotiating fees with doctors on a daily basis, why shouldn't individual consumers do so? Even a fully insured consumer should think about negotiating fees when it seems appropriate. I often negotiate a no-fee, follow-up visit with a doctor when its sole purpose is to check out if something done weeks prior is working. If nothing is found on the follow-up visit, I pay no fee. By so doing, I not only save my copayment or deductible but also save money for my insurer. And we all know where insurance money ultimately comes from.

Negotiating need not be limited to doctors. Consumers should also negotiate with health maintenance organizations and hospitals. Most HMOs are relatively new to the business. They may be part of a big insurance company, but few HMOs have operated for more than a handful of years. As a result, many issues arise for which the HMO has no policy. In those cases, which are surprisingly quite frequent, it is important to negotiate an acceptable outcome with the managed care company.

Every HMO is required by law to have an appeals process for consumer members who are not satisfied with a plan's decision. The appeals process is actually a negotiating session. You, and possibly your doctor, argue your point, and the managed care company argues its side. Then the two sides try to work out an agreement—one that is acceptable to both parties. From my experience, consumers who present a good, logical case usually win their appeal—meaning they negotiated a solution acceptable to everyone.

Several years ago, I helped a family whose child needed a very technically complex operation. The family had researched the procedure and discovered that a surgeon in Pittsburgh, Pennsylvania, was considered the most experienced in performing it on children. In fact, he operated on an average of 50 kids a year, using the exact procedure prescribed for this child.

A problem arose when the family's HMO, located more than 200 miles away from Pittsburgh, refused the family's request to take their child to this renowned surgeon. Instead, the HMO referred the young boy to a local surgeon who had only performed the surgery three times in his entire career. The family members were beside themselves. They couldn't afford to pay for the operation—with a cost upward of $40,000—out of their own pockets if they went to Pittsburgh on their own.

I suggested that the family negotiate a deal with the HMO. But I told them that first they had to prepare their case. That meant putting together a packet of information about the operation and about the surgeon in Pittsburgh, along with as much supporting material as possible. They did their homework. In a matter of two days, they had not only assembled the materials they had previously collected but also collected letters from the Pittsburgh surgeon, their own HMO primary care doctor and from the director of a self-help organization that helps parents of children with their child's condition. It was a very impressive packet of materials.

A meeting was set up with the local medical director of the HMO. In just five minutes, he agreed to the family's request.

So what had happened to change the HMO's mind in five minutes? First, by putting together all the facts in a logical case, the family made it easy for the medical director to see the options. Second—and here's where the family really made points—they argued that it would be more cost effective for the HMO to send the child to Pittsburgh. To have the surgery performed by the most skilled surgeon instead of a relative rookie was a much stronger guarantee of having a successful outcome. Further, they noted that the hospital in Pittsburgh was far more experienced in working with children with the condition, thus bringing greater expertise to the aftercare that would be necessary. In other words, they made the economic argument that having something done right the first time is a lot cheaper than having to pay the cost of possible mistakes.

The medical director was no dummy. That's why it only took five minutes.

I'm happy to report that the surgery went without a hitch. The HMO later made a deal with both that surgeon and the Pittsburgh hospital. In the future, any other children needing that operation would use their services.

So my doctor-critic is wrong in opposing the idea of con-sumer-practitioner negotiation. Just like in business, a good negotiation usually ends up with both sides winning. And frankly, I think negotiating for my health is a lot more impor-tant than negotiating any business deal I've ever entered into.

Getting
the Most
From
Managed
Care

⌒

Not long ago, I gave a speech to a hall full of union members. I talked about managed care—you know, health maintenance organizations and the like. A man in the audience stood up and said he would have nothing to do with managed care—ever. But when I asked him about his current insurance, I discovered he was enrolled in managed care without even knowing it. And the fact is, so are millions of other Americans.

Like my union friend's policy, if your health insurance policy requires that you get prior approval for a test, treatment or operation, that's managed care. If your employer provides coverage for medications but specifies certain pharmacies where the prescriptions must be filled, that's managed care. If your insurance covers hospitalization for mental illness but limits it to a certain number of days, that, too, is managed care. In other words, anytime your health insurance limits your choices, provides you with incentives (such as no out-of-pocket payment) to use certain providers or dictates where you can go for care, you are a part of managed care.

It may not have been your decision to belong to a managed care program, but here are some tips on getting the most out of your managed care plan.

Start by selecting the primary care doctor you want. Interview several from the managed care company's list. Choose the doctor that best meets your needs. If possible, conduct these interviews before you enroll in the managed care program. Make sure that whomever you choose is able to accept new patients. Sometimes, even though a practitioner's name is on the list, her practice is full.

Make sure you know all the plan's rules. For example, when does your plan allow you to seek a second opinion? This varies from plan to plan. If the answer is unclear from the literature you've been given, call the customer service number of your carrier and ask for the policy in writing. The company must provide it to you.

Find out how the appeals process in your managed care program works. This may sound technical, but it is absolutely vital that you know how to challenge decisions that you or your doctor don't agree with. Every managed care company is required to have an appeals process for services denied. Make sure you know it, and make sure you know how to use it.

And don't rely on your doctor to automatically act as

your go-between. Remember: She is also employed by, or under contract to, the managed care company. The greater the expenses the doctor runs up and the more trouble the doctor makes, the more likely it is that the doctor will not be working for, or kept under contract to, the managed care company for very long.

If things go wrong or you are dissatisfied with the program, complain to the customer service department of the managed care company. If you are enrolled through your employer, let the personnel director and company owner know about your problem. They talk to the managed care company's representative often and get quick resolutions to complaints. If you are enrolled in a Medicare HMO, file a complaint with your congressperson, as well as with the Medicare authorities, whom you can contact through your local Social Security office. Most managed care companies are very sensitive to customer complaints since they are trying to sell their services to as many people as possible.

Being in a managed care program is not like being in custody. Don't be afraid to exercise your rights and make your views known. Remember: You are the customer, and managed care is there to serve you.

Taking
Control

"What you're going to like about this class," the professor began, "is all the fighting that goes on!"

That's how my college class in dispute resolution started. And let me tell you, fight we did. Our teacher, a canny philosophy professor, never gave a lecture. Instead, he would divide the class into two groups, pose a problem and ask each group to argue opposing solutions. By the end of class, through negotiation, arbitration, coin toss or whatever, we had to reach some kind of an agreement.

The course was going well until one day near the end of the semester. The class could not come to an agreement. And frankly, both sides were upset.

"What do we do now?" we asked.

Our professor quietly came to the front of the classroom and told us we had just learned an important lesson. There are, he said, some problems for which the information needed to solve them is so contradictory, no single resolution will do. In those instances, the professor went on, people just have to make their own decisions about how to proceed.

I've been thinking about all this ever since a federal panel, put together by the National Cancer Institute, reported in January 1997 that it could not come to agreement about when women should start receiving routine mammograms.

This has been a controversial issue for a long time. The medical evidence clearly shows that mammography is an effective screening tool for cancer once a woman turns 50. It's also clear that women under 50 with a family history of breast cancer benefit, as well.

But it's not clear if mammograms are worthwhile for women under 50 who aren't at high risk. Studies have yet to determine if the odds of women in this group having a breast tumor detected are great enough to justify the intervention, some minimal exposure to radiation, the risk of an unnecessary biopsy and the expense of the yearly exam. As a result, recommendations varied. The American Cancer Society recommended mammograms every two years for women ages 40 to 49, and the NCI only recommended routine mammograms to women over age 50.

In the end, the federal panel abstained from making a recommendation. And the idea that women under 50 would be left with no clear directive on this issue, which was how the panel essentially left things in that January 1997 report, sent other groups into a tizzy.

A major uproar ensued. Many women's health advocates argued that it's better to be safe than sorry. They wanted the federal panel to change its recommendations. Many doctors and scientists felt there was just not enough evidence to warrant new standards. And of course, Congress got into the act. Several members threatened to hold hearings on the subject.

In March 1997, an American Cancer Society committee looked at the same evidence and nixed its own recommendation of a mammogram every other year for 40-to-49-year-old women in favor of a recommendation for an annual test.

Pretty soon, the National Cancer Institute capitulated

and changed its recommendation to include mammograms every other year for women ages 40 to 49. There was no new evidence. The studies were still as murky and contradictory as ever. But it was clear the NCI didn't have much choice. This battle had become not just a media event but a political event, as well.

Obviously, this was not your typical case of consensus building. The recommendation the NCI ultimately made was one that was forced upon it. Obviously, we know that the expert panel did not agree with the American Cancer Society panel. So as consumers, we're still left out in the cold. Apparently, this is what my philosophy professor meant when he said there are times when we have to use our own intelligence and interpretive powers when making a decision.

Surprisingly, this is often the case in health care. More often than not, there is no unanimous agreement on the best way to treat or deal with a medical problem. Hysterectomy is a perfect example. Only one out of every 10 hysterectomies performed stands up to a second opinion. In other words, about 90 percent of the time, doctors cannot agree if a particular hysterectomy is necessary. But does that mean a woman shouldn't have a hysterectomy if doctors disagree? Not necessarily. Practitioners are looking at clinical reasons why a hysterectomy should or should not be performed. But clinical analysis usually doesn't take into consideration the actual problem a woman is having. Sure, most women may not need hysterectomies to live long lives. But many women want them in order to live more comfortable lives. Does that make it wrong?

Or how about hormone replacement therapy? The studies are ever-changing on its benefits and risks. Gynecologists and medical researchers are often in radical disagreement over when and if the treatment is appropriate. Sure, women have gone through menopause without the therapy since time began. But is that a reason for not using a therapy? For women truly suffering from symptoms associated with menopause, HRT might be just the answer to improving and enhancing their lives. Do medical debates need to be settled before a person makes a choice? If that were the case, we'd still be treating infections with bleeding.

Most consumers are afraid to make their own medical decisions. We've been conditioned to think we are unable to analyze the data, to understand what a medical study or report means. We tend to rely on our doctors, who are often just as unsure or confused by conflicting studies. And often the reason a doctor might recommend something is not in concert with the patient's lifestyle or personal value system.

The bottom line here is that we need to think for ourselves. Clearly, there are sound data and consensus about the effects of smoking and obesity. One cannot argue with the benefits of wearing an automobile seat belt. But when the studies conflict, when there is no real consensus, it is up to all of us as individuals to look at the data and make decisions that are most beneficial to us.

Conflicting medical data should not be the basis for doing nothing. That's the easy way out, and it could be quite harmful. Indeed, conflicting information means each consumer has to work a little harder. Time will be necessary to review the information carefully. But if that is done, people will most likely make the decisions that are right for them.

And that is truly taking charge of one's own health.

PART III

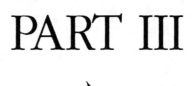

How
Can
That Be?

It's hard not to be cynical when you see so much fraud and abuse going on in the health care system. And every day, I am more amazed at how something even more incredible comes to my attention. But the fact is that each incident, story or study that surfaces usually affects unsuspecting health care consumers.

In the pages that follow, I discuss some of the things that have not only amazed me in recent years but have also really accelerated my advocacy instincts. Situations such as these are making most health care consumers suspect the motives and competence of our health care practitioners and leaders.

Protecting
Yourself

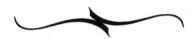

How unusual was March 1995? Headlines blared the story of a Florida man who had the wrong foot amputated in a Tampa hospital. A week later, a staff member at the same hospital mistakenly disconnected the respirator of a person on life support, causing an unwarranted death. In the Midwest, a surgeon performing a mastectomy removed the wrong breast. And in Boston, it was revealed that staff at the Dana-Farber Cancer Institute, one of the foremost cancer research facilities and hospitals, had mistakenly—and fatally—overdosed the *Boston Globe*'s health reporter with an experimental drug used in the treatment of breast cancer.

These were not headlines in sleazy tabloids. These were in papers ranging from the *New York Times* to the *Christian Science Monitor.* They were reports that raised wrenching questions about the quality of American hospitals and of the health care system in general.

Some medical professionals called these incidents unusual. And as they did with the spate of fatal airplane crashes in 1994, authorities raced forward to assure the public that these goofs were isolated incidents in a safe world.

But should we be reassured? The answer is no. In 1991, a Harvard study estimated that 86,000 people a year *die* from negligence in American hospitals. A study in a 1997 issue of the *Lancet* suggested that the true number is at least three times that amount. Hundreds of thousands more are permanently injured or maimed. Ten thousand people a year die from anesthesia-related mishaps. The director of the infection control section of the Centers for Disease Control and Prevention estimates that 80,000 people die from nosocomial (hospital-caused) infections each year. He estimates that one-third could be prevented.

To some people, these statistics are surprising. Haven't we made miraculous advances in the treatment of medical problems over the past few decades? Hasn't the new and improved technology that we've heard so much about made a significant difference in surgical and medical outcomes? How can hospitals be getting worse, as these studies suggest, when all we hear is how they're getting better?

Let's start with the improvements. There's no question that technology and new medical techniques have been a blessing to most consumers. Operations such as the coronary bypass procedure or the laparoscopic gallbladder removal have saved and improved the lives of millions of people. New medications have allowed people to improve the quality of their lives for years—even while they're suffering from chronic, often debilitating conditions.

But these new techniques and breakthroughs have had an unexpected side effect. They have reduced the demand for hospital beds, making the average hospital half empty on any given day and forcing those facilities to cut corners when it comes to costs. As a result, consumer safety can easily decline. People can fall through the cracks. A pruned and overextended staff will make mistakes. In fact, most hospitals have reduced the number of registered nurses, the quality backbone of the hospital, replacing them with personnel with less training, some of whom have less than a month's worth of education.

Of course, hospitals argue that even with the decline in demand and the cutbacks in highly trained personnel, consumer safety has not been jeopardized. But studies seem to contradict their proclamations. In fact, the nosocomial infection rate I discussed earlier has doubled in the last 15 years. And while there is no doubt that today's hospitals have patients far sicker than the typical hospital did 15 years ago, that is still no justification for a doubling of the infection rate.

I've also heard hospital personnel blame patients for these horrendous outcomes. But that's merely a diversionary tactic—one designed to take the responsibility off their own shoulders. I've met and spoken with Willie King, the Florida man who had the wrong foot amputated. He did absolutely nothing wrong—except trust the people at the hospital. He is a kind, gentle and bright individual. Blaming him or most other victims of medical incompetence is simply passing the buck.

I also knew Betsy Lehman of the *Boston Globe*. She interviewed me on several occasions for stories she was working on. If ever there was a savvy medical consumer, she was it. And from all accounts, she knew there was something wrong almost right away. But her protests fell on the deaf ears of arrogant medical professionals who apparently considered the consumer unable to sense a problem.

What happened in March 1995 is happening every month, but without the national publicity. People are being injured and neglected in American hospitals too often. Much of this could be prevented if hospitals really paid attention to the competence of their staffs and the quality of their care. Yet this may be a long time in the offing. In the meantime, as individual consumers, we must take charge of our own care.

What can you do to protect yourself from becoming a hospital casualty? First, ask questions. If you're considering surgery, find out how many times your doctor has performed the appropriate procedure in the last year. Ask the same question about the hospital. The more often a procedure has been performed, the better. Compare the rate with that of other doctors and facilities. Don't let reputations and bedside manner get in the way of hard facts. Ask about the hospital's overall infection rate, and find out the rate for your specific procedure. Also, get them to tell you the drug error rate at the facility. While most hospitals do not want to reveal this information, all of them keep it. Insist on finding out.

Once you are admitted to the hospital, be watchful. Don't be afraid to have a family member or friend with you at all times if you are too ill to advocate for yourself. Say no to things that do not seem right—such as the offering of a pill different than the one they normally bring—until such discrepancies are cleared up. Don't be afraid to speak up. Studies show that patients who ask questions leave the hospital quicker and in better health than their less assertive counterparts.

Of course, doctors and nurses are only human. They will make mistakes. But you can do plenty to cut down your chances of a hospital error happening to you.

Up in Smoke?

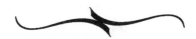

I'm a guy who loves politics. In many ways, I'm a political junkie. I read political magazines, watch all the Sunday morning news programs and really get into watching liberal and conservative pundits go at it on shows such as *Crossfire*. When I was a kid in grammar school, I knew the name of every United States senator and most of the members of the House of Representatives.

So there's really not much that surprises or confuses me when it comes to politicians.

But in 1997, I must admit, I was extremely confused. And it all had to do with what Congress was doing about the issue of kids' health and tobacco. At the time, things that I was reading in newspapers and watching on television made no sense to me at all. Plus, I was having this alarming recurring dream. And frankly, I thought I was confusing fantasy with reality.

Let me explain.

My confusion started when liberal Senator Ted Kennedy from Massachusetts teamed up with conservative Senator Orrin Hatch of Utah to introduce legislation that would raise federal taxes on cigarettes. Did I hear right? Kennedy and Hatch cosponsoring a bill? And Hatch supporting a tax increase? Well, I thought, Kennedy has sure tricked old Orrin on that one.

In fact, I liked the tax increase idea. If you make the price of cigarettes excessively expensive, you discourage people, especially kids, from smoking them. And that's good.

But just when I thought I had it figured out, I learned that the money generated from the tax would pay for health care for up to 10 million American kids who have no health insurance.

Wait a minute, I thought. If you're going to use cigarette taxes to pay for kids' health, but the idea of the tax is to stop people from smoking, how can the program be successful? I mean, if the tax works, fewer people will be buying cigarettes. And if there are fewer people smoking, there won't be enough money to pay for the health insurance these kids need. And to add to the confusion, if the tax doesn't reduce the number of smokers, we'll need to find a new tax to pay for all the illnesses those smokers get over their lifetimes.

Are you starting to understand why I was so confused?

But hold on. Let me tell you about that recurring dream I was having.

I'm driving along a highway when I see a billboard with the infamous Joe Camel coyly staring out at me. Next to him is a pack of cigarettes with a picture of a little boy lying in an oxygen tent. Senators Kennedy and Hatch are standing next to the boy, each with reassuring smiles. And under this heartwarming scene, written in huge words, is this caption: HELP AMERICA'S CHILDREN—START SMOKING TODAY!

I tell you I was going crazy. Of course, it's good public policy to discourage smoking. And it's also good to want to help innocent children get the medical care they need. But it seems to me the Kennedy-Hatch plan was a contradiction. If it worked, it failed because as soon as tobacco sales decreased, poor kids would suffer.

And why had these two admired senators ignored President Clinton's proposal? He, too, proposed a health insurance program for uninsured children and an increase in the federal cigarette tax. But his proposal didn't link the two together. His plan guaranteed that America's poor kids would get health insurance even if every smoker went cold turkey tomorrow.

Actually, talking this all out and the benefit of time have helped me a lot. I now realize it's not me who was confused—it was those politicians in Washington. If they were really against smoking, they would have just stopped sending us mixed messages. Maybe then our respect for leaders would start to climb.

Greed

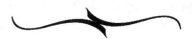

You would think it was 1929, the start of the Great Depression, if you were to hear the comments I received from doctors a few years ago when it was reported that their overall income dropped by 4 percent in 1994.

"How do you expect us to maintain quality if we have to fight for the next buck?" one irate specialist asked me.

"This is the beginning of the end for medicine as we know it," a 40-year medical veteran said.

"I'm thinking about looking into another profession," said a doctor in his early 30s.

Before you get out your crying towel, let's put this whole thing into perspective. First of all, even with the drop, the average doctor's income in 1994 was $187,000. It's remained pretty much the same since then, as well. But that's take-home pay! Doctors in the subspecialties of internal medicine, surgery and pediatrics took home more than $240,000. And that doesn't count income they often receive from side businesses they own, such as physical therapy centers and diagnostic labs.

But the whining from the medical community over the drop just wouldn't stop. A young female doctor, in her first year of practice, complained she only earned $85,000. Sure, she had $50,000 in education debts and had to go through five years of a low-paying residency, but I'd like her to meet some of my schoolteacher friends who have as many years of education and will never earn $85,000.

Experts were quick to point out the reasons for the decline in doctors' pay. Some blamed managed care, which has forced doctors to charge less for their services. The managed care industry, though, said the drop in income came about because the United States has a glut of doctors—particularly specialists.

Others said the drop coincided with a rise in group practices. Such practices allow docs to work fewer hours and therefore earn less.

Managed care, the national excess of doctors and the growth of group practices have led to a decline in income. And since all these trends are expected to continue, it's likely that physician income will decline further in years to come.

But the real question is, should we care? Does the decline in doctor earnings mean we will see a decline in medical quality? If medicine is no longer the road to riches, as it has been for the last 40 years, will we see fewer bright students entering the profession?

Frankly, I don't think we have too much to worry about. There is no sign that lower physician incomes have in any way decreased medical quality. And there are no signs that they will. Let's face it: When an anesthesiologist's income drops from $224,000 in 1993 to $214,000 in 1994, that's not a crisis.

Nor should we worry about attracting high-caliber students to medical school. There's no indication that's becoming a problem. In truth, I'd rather young people be attracted to medicine for the right reason again—to treat people, not to treat themselves to infinite riches.

No, for my money—which is not anywhere near their money—I think the shakeout in physician income is a good sign. And if the doctors I spoke to don't like it, let them quit. They probably won't be serving their patients well anyway if they're constantly worrying about where their next Mercedes will come from.

Who's Benefiting?

I'm sure you'll find this hard to believe, but consider what happened to me when I first heard the news of insurance giant Aetna buying managed care giant U.S. Healthcare back in 1996.

"I have a long-distance, person-to-person collect call for Mr. Charles Inlander," the operator said.

"Who's calling?" I asked.

"It's Mother Teresa," she responded. "Calling from India."

I gladly accepted the charges.

"Hello, Mother Teresa. What an honor it is for me to talk to you! What can I do for you?"

"Well, Mr. Inlander, maybe you can explain something to me."

"Of course. What is it you'd like to know?"

"Last week, a sister visited me from the United States. She told me that a big American insurance company was buying a large managed care company for $8.9 billion. Could that be true?"

"You must mean the Aetna Life and Casualty Company purchasing U.S. Healthcare," I said. "Yes, that's true."

"Isn't that a lot of money? I mean, if the company is worth $8.9 billion, U.S. Healthcare must serve at least half the U.S. population!"

"Well, not really, Mother," I informed her. "Actually, U.S. Healthcare has fewer than 3 million subscribers, and of course, they don't see all of them every year. But speaking of a lot of money, one man, U.S. Healthcare's chief executive officer, is going to receive $900 million of the purchase price in cash and stock."

"I'm sorry," she said. "I think our connection is bad. How much did you say that man is getting?"

"Nine hundred million dollars in cash and stock," I repeated.

There was a long silence on the other end of the phone.

"You know, Mr. Inlander," she went on, "maybe you all are getting used to these amounts, but how could one man need $900 million? In India, that would vaccinate millions of children, pay for hundreds of thousands of surgeries and save tens of thousands of lives."

"It certainly is a lot of money," I agreed quietly.

"But tell me something else, then," she asked. "How much do people pay to be covered by U.S. Healthcare?"

"Last year," I told her, "U.S. Healthcare collected $3.6 billion in premiums."

"Oh, I see," she said. "So $3.6 billion was what they spent on medical care?"

"Not really," I responded. "U.S. Healthcare is a very efficient company. They only had to spend 75 percent of that amount on medical care. That's partly why Aetna wanted to buy them."

"That does sound good," she said. "That means they had about $1.4 billion left over to use this year. Did they drop this year's premiums by 25 percent?"

"It doesn't work like that, Mother. Some of that money

went to pay for the administrative costs of the company. For example, the man I told you would be getting $900 million in cash and stock was also paid several million in salary and bonuses. Other officials were paid high salaries, as well. After administrative costs, $381 million was left over in profit. That's what goes to the shareholders."

"So you're telling me that in the United States, it's a good thing if only 75 cents of every premium dollar actually goes for health care?"

"That's right. That's the American way."

"I must say, Mr. Inlander, it's all too confusing, and I've kept you on the phone a long time. Thank you for your help. And by the way, if you know anyone who has some extra bandages or unused medications, we could sure use them."

Just then the alarm clock roared in my ear. The whole conversation had been a dream. Yet even now, I can't help wonder what it will take before we all come out of this stupor and wake up to how increasingly greedy and self-serving the American health care system has become.

Deadly Souvenirs

On that day in 1996 when the Valu-Jet plane crashed in the Florida Everglades, killing more than 110 people, at least 220 people died from infections they acquired in the hospital! The next day, not a single plane went down. However, 220 more people died from hospital-acquired infections, fancily called nosocomial infections.

I draw these comparisons not to diminish the Valu-Jet tragedy, but to point out a less-publicized tragedy that we should also find disturbing. And there is no mystery as to its cause.

The number one reason that people in hospitals pick up other people's bugs is that medical personnel do not wash their hands. That's right. It's that stupid and simple. But increasingly, it's not surprising.

Studies show, for instance, that only half of all doctors actually wash their hands between patient examinations. The stats on nurses aren't much better.

And despite protests to the contrary, hospitals don't take infection control seriously. They pay lip service to infection standards issued by the Centers for Disease Control and Prevention, but rarely do they have adequate infection control programs in place. Nor do they put the financial resources into maintaining a significant program.

Part of what's so outrageous about the situation is that hospitals spend tens of thousands of dollars each year on new technology. They tout their MRI machines or talk up their latest laser surgery that gets you in and out of the hospital in hours rather than days. But they have not invested in the basics, such as courses in hand washing. Maybe it's too mundane.

Or maybe there is money to be made on infections. I'm not suggesting that hospitals deliberately give people infections or are lax on infection control for monetary gain. However, I am troubled by the fact that patients who come down with infections do generate more revenue for hospitals. In other words, now that fewer people are entering hospitals for fewer days, could there be a perverse incentive to keep them there longer? I don't know.

What I do know is that by the end of this year, 80,000 Americans will die from infections they got in the hospital. And this will occur despite overwhelming medical consensus that half—fully half—of these infections can be prevented.

So what can be done? Plenty. First, all hospitals should be required to meet the Centers for Disease Control and Prevention's infection guidelines. Every hospital should have a *trained, full-time* infection control officer on staff. Hospitals should also have to report their nosocomial infections to state health departments, which, in turn, should have to share that information with federal authorities. And every hospital should be required to publicize nosocomial infection rates annually. There are no such requirements today! In fact, if it were up to me, every hospital would have a neon sign in front of its entrance listing the percentage of people currently in the hospital who have acquired one of these deadly souvenirs. I'd wager that the number of infections would drop by half if this became standard practice!

We, as consumers, must be more vigilant, too. If you or a loved one is hospitalized, don't let doctors or nurses—or any other hospital personnel—touch you without washing their hands. If the doctor or nurse comes in wearing gloves, make him put new ones on in your room. If you see hospital personnel—from food service workers to candy stripers—not washing their hands between patient contacts, mention it to their supervisors.

There's a quip among medical people that a hospital is the worst place to put a sick person. Ha ha! Maybe it's time to put that joke to rest.

White-Coat Crime

Two weeks after my daughter was born in 1982, I received a bill from the hospital. The total charge: just over $3,000. As I reviewed the itemized invoice, though, I realized that there were many mistakes. For example, my wife and I were charged for use of a delivery room we never used. There were also charges for two visits by a pediatrician we never saw and for drugs my wife never received. The errors were significant: They comprised one-third of the bill.

I immediately called the hospital and was told by a billing clerk that I shouldn't worry about the mistakes—my insurance company had already paid its 80 percent of the charges. I would be billed for the rest. I called my insurer, who promised to look into it. When I heard nothing from the company, I called back. I was told there was no record of my complaint. I told the insurer that unless this invoice was corrected, I would report the matter to the state's attorney general. Two days later, I received a call from the vice president of my insurance company, who told me "in confidence" that the matter had been resolved. And as a favor to me, he was waiving my copayment. I doubt they ever collected a dime from the hospital—or even tried.

In the mid-1980s, things began to change... a little. Public audits showed high rates of hospital billing errors and, at the very least, pointed to something terribly wrong. The problem was that Republican administrations tended to ignore the findings. However, when Bill Clinton took office and health care was *numero uno* on his agenda, the impact that fraudulent and sloppy hospital billing was having on the federal treasury suddenly got the attention it deserved.

The year 1996 was a good example. Two prestigious not-for-profit hospitals in Philadelphia paid a total of $42 million in fines and reimbursements for wrongfully billing Medicare. By 1997, the for-profit hospital chain Columbia/HCA had been nabbed for its billing practices. More than 4,000 of the nation's 6,000 hospitals were also being investigated for overbilling government programs, and federal officials uncovered data that showed the home care industry abusing the system in a big way.

Hospitals argue that they're being singled out for innocent errors and that Medicare and Medicaid rules are too complicated and convoluted. They claim that if rules were clearer and easier to follow, mistakes would rarely occur. Hospitals, in fact, got so caught up in this view that in July 1997, the president of the American Hospital Association sent a letter to President Clinton asking for a six-month moratorium on new investigations. He told Clinton that hospital officials "...feel there's a system of extortion in place here." The administration wasn't moved by this analogy, and the request was denied.

Hallelujah!

It's pretty incredible that it took the government so long to go after these white-coat criminals. As far back as 1984, reports were being released showing that more than 90 percent of all hospital bills had errors in them. One audit reported in 1984 by the Equifax Corporation, covering numerous hospitals bills of $10,000 or more, found that 98 percent had errors. And 75 percent of the errors were in favor of the hospital, with the average error being approximately $1,400. Over the years, private insurers have been inundated by calls from policyholders who questioned charges submitted by doctors and hospitals. But most consumers report that their protests fell on deaf ears.

Health care providers like to hold themselves above the fray. And years ago, they probably were. In those days, the local physician was likely to be the best-educated person in town. People not only turned to him for medical care but also for general advice. Doctors were respected. And they earned that respect by being there when people needed them, caring for the rich and poor and putting in long, grueling hours.

As a child growing up in Chicago in the 1950s, I remember how dedicated our family doctor was. Day or night you could call him—he gladly gave us his home phone number (a rarity today!). He made house calls. I never went to his office when I was sick; he came to see me. He always looked tired. And he was. But wouldn't you be if you were going out to visit patients at all hours? And I can assure you that he wasn't rich. In fact, I'm sure many people couldn't pay him for his services, and I know he would accept a dinner in lieu of his fee.

I am not trying to wax nostalgic here. I'm simply comparing his style with that of our modern health care providers. And I am not suggesting that he was more competent than today's practitioners. I'm sure he wasn't.

But old Dr. Cohen would never think of overcharging a patient or submitting an inflated bill. I know it never occurred to him that he should set his fees to accommodate the lifestyle he wanted to live. No, he lived a lifestyle that reflected what his patients could afford to pay. And that was pretty modest. He wasn't going to gouge his patients. And I know for a fact that he would stop by to see how a patient was getting along for many weeks after a treatment without ever charging for a follow-up visit.

Clearly, that has changed. Too many of our health care providers today believe that they deserve a certain style of living. They view their medical licenses as certificates to the good life rather than as permission to serve. As a result, most doctors shun patients without insurance, restrict the number of Medicaid patients they accept and think nothing of charging exorbitant fees for what are clearly minimal services.

Physicians and hospital administrators are angry these days. They're upset that professional life isn't what it used to be. Simply translated, what they want is the ability to do whatever they want without anybody questioning their decisions or looking over their shoulders. That's what hospitals are saying when they write President Clinton, asking him to hold off on federal investigations of billing errors. And that's what older doctors are saying when they advise their children not to go into medicine. Now that the screen of accountability is hanging over health care, many professionals just don't like practicing anymore.

When I had my run-in with hospital billing practices, it was obvious that no one but me cared. But that's changing as both private insurers and the government are making concerted efforts to carefully review expenditures and prosecute the bad guys. And I'm confident this trend will continue.

It's about time.

My Advice? Get Into Prostates

Dustin Hoffman's character in the 1960s movie *The Graduate* was pulled aside at a party and confidentially advised to "get into plastics." The idea, of course, was that there was a great deal of money to be made in the plastics business, and if he got into it, he was bound to be a rich man later.

Well, if I were advising a young person today about a way to make big bucks, I'd say, "Get into prostates!"

Just so everyone knows what we're talking about here, the prostate gland is not a sex organ, as many people think, but it does have a lot to do with sexual reproduction. Located at the base of the bladder, it secretes a fluid that helps support and nourish sperm.

As men get older, problems can occur with the prostate. Half of all American men develop enlarged prostates that affect urination. And one in five will develop prostate cancer, with 41,000 dying from it each year. In fact, the prostate gland causes more misery for men than just about any other structure in the body, and sexual performance is the least of those problems.

For years, there have been effective treatments for enlarged prostates—not so for prostate cancer. And while prostate cancer has become more easily diagnosed, mainly due to the prostate-specific antigen blood test, the medical establishment has also *claimed* great progress in effectively treating the disease by coming up with all sorts of controversial techniques.

Topping the list is an operation called the radical prostatectomy, or total surgical removal of the prostate gland. In 1990, this operation was so infrequently performed that it didn't even rank in the 100 most-performed surgeries in the United States. By 1996, it had shot up to number four.

And the evidence suggests this enormous jump is due to greed more than to medical need. Consider these facts.

Radical surgery for prostate cancer has not been proven to be a lifesaver, especially for men over the age of 70. In 1997, nevertheless, 250,000 of those men had the operation, which often results in all sorts of side effects, with infection, impotence and incontinence being among the most common.

And it should come as no surprise that the radical prostatectomy is the most expensive of all prostate cancer treatments. As one surgical professor observed to me, "If Medicare paid a surgeon $500 for the operation, instead of thousands, I doubt most men over 70 would have it recommended to them."

Women have been dealt this "greed-equals-need" equation for years with unnecessary hysterectomies and cesarean sections. Now men have a procedure all their own to contend with, replete with national warnings about prostate cancer, advertisements featuring famous generals and Hollywood stars, and television talk shows devoted to this walnut-sized gland.

As a result, most of us men are scared to death of our prostate gland. When something goes wrong, we start thinking of a last will and testament rather than our options. And that's where we make our mistake. Instead of yielding to unnecessary surgery or racing to the latest unproven herbal remedy, we should be seeking second opinions and more information. The facts about prostate disease, including cancer, are not hard to find. Armed with them, men can assure themselves of getting the most effective treatment and the best results.

It's hard to imagine that such a tiny little gland could stir up so much controversy. But business is business, and medicine has always gone where the money is.

A
Bitter Pill
to Swallow

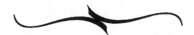

Today, more than 46,000 Americans will walk out of their local pharmacy with either the wrong prescription medication or the wrong dosage. Tomorrow, the same number of mistakes will be made. And over the course of the next year, 17 million people will be given the wrong prescription by a pharmacist.

The consequences of these mistakes can be devastating. At least 20 percent of people admitted to hospitals are there because of a problem with their medication—perhaps a mistake made at the pharmacy or an improper drug ordered by a doctor. Some have had an unexpected reaction to a medication. Many of those people would be home and well if a prescription error had not been made. Other victims may never enter a hospital, but they don't get better, either. If doctors don't suspect a prescription error, they're apt to misdiagnose, which leads to more mistakes.

What's happened to create this situation? Why are pharmacy error rates going up? Aren't pharmacists better trained than ever? And aren't there government agencies overseeing all this?

One problem is the sheer volume of medications now being prescribed. More than 2.5 billion prescriptions were filled in the United States last year, according to the U.S. Food and Drug Administration. And that is expected to increase by 10 percent this year. The more medications being dispensed, the more opportunity for error.

Another problem has to do with the growth of drug-store chains. Some pharmacy associations claim that chains are trying to increase profits by cutting back on the number of pharmacists they employ. Fewer pharmacists handling a growing number of prescriptions creates another potent combination for mistakes. In fact, the North Carolina Pharmacy Board enacted a rule limiting the number of prescriptions a single pharmacist can fill in a day. The intent is to cut back on errors. But most state boards, which are supposed to be protecting the public, have not taken any action, leading advocates such as myself to think that it may require direct legislative action to protect consumers who use retail drugstores.

As for whether pharmacists are making mistakes because they weren't trained properly, I don't think that's the real issue. Pharmacists really don't do much delicate mixing of ingredients behind the counter anymore: Today, they're mostly pouring pills from large containers into smaller jars and bottles.

This means that the onus of safety is falling onto the backs of consumers. Yet most of us know little about medications. Pills look alike. Most have no easily identifiable marks on them that give us the kind of information we need to know if we've been given the wrong pill. Even our doctors are little help. I've spoken to several doctors who've quietly told me that they couldn't tell one pill from another simply by looking.

Once again, greed is threatening consumer safety. As these big drugstore chains cut back on pharmacists to cut costs, they are risking the lives of their customers. Back in the late 1980s, my father-in-law had a long-standing prescription refilled at his local drugstore. He'd been taking the same pills for years. His druggist had always had another pharmacist working with him. But because of the pressure of chain store competition, he was forced to cut the other pharmacist's hours. He just couldn't afford him full-time. When my father-in-law got the prescription home, my mother-in-law noticed that the pills were a different color. She had the wherewithal to call the pharmacy and ask for a size and color description of the pill. Bottom line—the pharmacist had given him the wrong medication. He explained that he was so busy that it just slipped by. Needless to say, that was the last time my in-laws used that pharmacy.

To be safe, you, as a health care consumer, must put in place a strategy to protect yourself from being a victim of these errors. First, you have to make sure you know exactly what drug you are supposed to receive. When the doctor writes out a prescription, ask him to translate the scribble. When you pick up a prescription, ask the pharmacist to double-check to make sure it's the right medication. This is even more important if the pharmacist is dispensing a generic product because it will probably have a different name than the one the doctor wrote down.

If it's a refill, compare the new contents with the old

ones. Are the pills the same color and size? Is the liquid a different consistency or smell?

And when in doubt about a drug received from a mail-order pharmacy, take it to a local store to be checked out. In this day and age, you shouldn't be afraid to ask questions of your pharmacist or any pharmacist. It may save your life.

Breaking
the Social
Contract

My mother was born at a public hospital in Chicago almost 90 years ago. Very few babies were born in hospitals back then, but my grandmother's brother, a young doctor, convinced her that both mother and newborn would have a better chance of survival if she used a hospital.

They chose a public hospital over a private hospital because it cost less—a lot less. Remember: There was no health insurance in those days. And my grandparents felt safer in a facility backed by the government. They had heard terrible stories about patients being neglected in many of the private, doctor-owned facilities that had begun to sprout up. Plus, back then, public hospitals were seen as part of the social contract the citizens of the United States had with their government and each other. This same social contract later led to the creation of many citizen-government programs such as Social Security, Medicare and Medicaid.

The circumstances of my mother's birth came to mind recently as I considered how determined most states are today to have their Medicaid populations (those low-income or disabled people enrolled in the public joint federal and state health insurance plan) receive their health care through private health maintenance organizations.

On the surface, the idea seems good for all involved. HMOs that want this business—and there are a growing number of them that do—contract with states to provide certain specified services for a set monthly fee. Companies calculate that even with the added expense of the many health problems that Medicaid recipients tend to have, HMOs can't do any worse than break even.

For people on Medicaid, such a plan would open the doors to health care they never before received. Access to health care is often difficult for Medicaid recipients because many private doctors never take Medicaid patients, while others limit Medicaid visits to a few hours a week. An HMO plan would also mean that Medicaid beneficiaries would not have to use a private hospital's emergency room for primary care—something most have been doing for years because it's often been the only option.

All in all, better primary care, more emphasis on prevention, more control over emergency room use and fixed fees—all trademarks of HMOs and managed care—should save money for the states. Plus, by turning over Medicaid to private HMOs, cities and counties can begin to sell off or close down their public clinics. Let the private sector run those, too.

It's a win-win situation for everyone, it seems. Or is it?

Maybe Medicaid HMOs will work in the short term, but I'm not too sure of their long-term viability. What happens when their profits start to drop? Will they still be able to provide the federally mandated services each Medicaid recipient is entitled to receive? Profits at most HMOs in the United States started declining in 1996, and by the end of 1997, almost 70 percent of the nation's HMOs were actually losing money.

There's a very high likelihood that Medicaid HMOs could go belly-up pretty quickly if states do not intervene by increasing the amount they're willing to pay for medical care. And that, of course, leads to an even bigger worry: Where will people go when a Medicaid HMO goes out of business? If public clinics and facilities truly disappear, who will take care of the people who rely on them?

It's easy to forget a bit of history. When Medicaid began in the mid-1960s, a lot of public hospitals closed because private hospitals started accepting the poor—now that they were insured. It seemed private hospitals welcomed the new revenue and government contracts and would do their best to treat the poor. But when the profits from Medicaid started to decline, mainly in the 1970s as health care costs rose faster than the government's Medicaid payments, lots of private hospitals shunned the responsibility.

By the late 1970s, stories began appearing in newspapers all across the country of poor people being denied needed medical services, despite the fact that most of them held Medicaid cards. Unfortunately, at the same time, medical inflation started zooming. By the early 1980s, the annual medical inflation rate was rising by as much as 14 or 15 percent. And while the Medicaid reimbursement levels to hospitals rose in those years, they did not rise as fast as inflation. As a result, private hospitals used every means available to fill their beds with the higher-paying patients, primarily employees working for companies offering very generous health plans.

Still another phenomenon was occurring. Try as they might to bring in patients, hospitals were actually seeing more and more of their beds going empty by the late 1980s. Technology, along with safe and less costly outpatient services, was taking business away from hospitals. By the 1990s, the majority of the people in hospitals were often the very sick and the very poor. The poor were often forced into hospitals because no private doctors would take them.

When the Medicaid program came into law, just a few years after Medicare, it was viewed as an extension of the social contract that the public had with the government. Between Medicare and Medicaid, the federal government promised us, the public, that our medical needs would be taken care of when we grew older or became impoverished. But as years went by and the financial pressures of health care became so significant, that contract began to be breeched. And it was especially easy to deny care to the poor, most of whom were unable to speak with influence in any social debate.

Which brings us back to Medicaid HMOs. Despite all the promises and assurances about how they will restore the public's faith in the government's promise to take care of the medical needs of the poor, the symptoms of failure are already starting to appear. Reports have shown that many states are being pressured by Medicaid HMOs to raise the level of reimbursement. There have even been news stories suggesting some Medicaid HMOs are in tight financial straits. It's just as clear as can be—the private sector is not going to be able to handle this problem. And it doesn't seem that our elected officials are ready to face the facts and be honest with all the citizens about what must be done.

My grandparents trusted the government over the private sector. In today's national mood, they'd be labeled politically naive. But the government delivered for them and, over the years, did so for millions of others. Public health care was always there when the private sector walked away. I only hope that it's there the next time doors shut to the poor.

A Message to Washington

"Hello, Mr. Inlander. The congressman asked me to call you. He thought you could give me the names of people who have been victims of managed care."

The caller was an assistant to a then first-term representative from Iowa.

"What do you mean 'victim'?" I asked.

"You know," she said. "People who have been hurt because health maintenance organizations have put gag orders on doctors. Or people who have died because they were denied an operation. You know, people like that."

"I'll tell you," I replied. "If a doctor has a gag order from an HMO, the consumer is highly unlikely to find out. And very few dead people have contacted me about being denied surgery. Why don't you tell me what you are trying to accomplish, and maybe I can help you."

"Well, the House Commerce Committee is going to hold hearings on managed care. The congressman is a member of that committee. He's looking for people to testify who have been harmed by managed care."

"Is there some specific legislation being considered?" I asked.

"Well, I'm not sure," she answered. "But he is looking for victims."

"What about people who are satisfied with managed care?" I inquired. "Do you think the congressman would like to have some of them testify?"

"I doubt it," she said. "He didn't ask for any."

"I see. I have one other question you can answer for me. Has the congressman introduced any health legislation since he came to Congress?"

"Why, no!" she replied somewhat startled. "He's interested in business. But if you have any ideas, maybe he will!"

Well, that about wrapped up our conversation, and although I didn't end up being very helpful, I wasn't surprised to receive a phone call like that.

Health legislation became all the rage when President Clinton was elected. And even though Clinton's health proposal was never passed, since then a whole slew of bills have been introduced, and some have been enacted into law. Some examples: A handful of states passed laws guaranteeing women at least two days in the hospital after delivering a baby, and the federal government soon did the same. In Congress, Senator Ted Kennedy and former Senator Nancy Kassebaum pushed through a law that ensures health insurance for people who switch jobs. In Pennsylvania, a state representative introduced legislation prohibiting nonregistered nurses from treating patients in the hospital; in Illinois, a bill would make medical records more private.

From all this activity, you would think that health care reform is at the top of the nation's legislative agenda. But think again. These bills, and thousands of more like them, are typical of legislation introduced every year at both the state and federal levels. And the vast majority, more than 90 percent, are never acted upon. Am I being too cynical? Well, you tell me.

Next to Social Security, members of Congress report receiving more mail about health care than any other subject. Some of the mail comes from senior citizens concerned about Medicare. But many letters spell out specific problems that constituents are having with the rapidly changing health care system. In response, legislators introduce legislation. Most of the time, they know very little about the subject. And more often than not, they do very little to make their bill become law.

But back home, they are health care champions. At town meetings, in constituent newsletters and in the local media, they tout themselves as defenders of the public's health by reciting all the bills they introduced or cosponsored.

I had never even heard of the congressman whose aide called me about the managed care hearings. I'm sure you haven't either. But elections were coming up that November, and this fellow, like many others, was up for reelection. He needed to show his constituency back in Iowa that he cares about their health. He jumped on the gag-order bandwagon because that topic was making a lot of headlines around the country at the time. It seems that many doctors were telling reporters that their contracts with HMOs were forcing them to withhold information from their patients.

I know that the congressman whose aide called me never saw a contract with such a gag rule in it. No one was able to produce one at any of the hearings held on the subject. And by 1997, after a very careful investigation, the federal government had been unable to find a single managed care contract that contained a gag rule.

What's obvious about all this is that too many times even some well-intentioned politicos go off ranting and raving about something they know nothing about. And it doesn't seem to bother them that often their actions push through unnecessary legislation or bad laws.

Well, it bothers me. And we should hold these esteemed members of our legislatures far more accountable.

PART IV

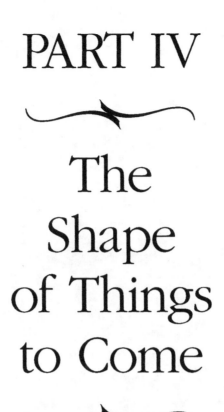

The
Shape
of Things
to Come

The future of health care is being driven by many interesting and complex factors. From technological advancements and scientific discoveries to cost pressures and consumer rights, the shape of tomorrow's health system will be very different from what we know today. And yet "tomorrow" is very much upon us as we struggle to blend the health care system we know with the one that is to be.

What follows are my views of some of the most important changes. While I am excited about what can be, I'm worried that greed, professional self-interest and misguided policy makers may slow down progress. And to me, progress is simply defined as what is best for the medical consumer.

Worrying About Medicare

As a 51-year-old baby boomer, I'm worried about Medicare. I'm concerned about my parents, both of whom are in their late 80s and rely heavily on Medicare benefits. I'm nervous that Congress may jiggle and juggle the Medicare books in such a way that my parents will become financially strapped if Washington goes too far in paring the Medicare budget.

But I have a personal interest, as well. I'm only 14 years away from being eligible for Medicare myself, and I'm beginning to wonder whether I can count on the program as the centerpiece of my health insurance. I'm also troubled by the thought that my 16-year-old daughter, Amy, may not have adequate health care when she reaches old age.

In 1997, the debate in Washington was how to save Medicare beyond the year 2002—that's when government actuaries originally estimated the Medicare Trust Fund would go bankrupt. Congress, if you recall, put a temporary Band-Aid on the problem by passing the 1997 Budget Act. That supposedly assures money in the fund until 2007.

But in reality, short-term fixes are not legislative issues at all. What is really before Congress and all the citizens of this country is how we will fund Medicare for the next 30, 40 and 50 years.

Here's what's at stake. Prior to the advent of Medicare, the majority of Americans 65 and older had no health insurance. Many people died prematurely because they could not afford basic medical services. Even in those days, when a day in the hospital cost less than $100, most senior citizens could not afford a prolonged illness. I remember when my 74-year-old grandfather got very sick in 1957. The whole family was making plans to bring him home because we could not afford many more days of hospitalization. My grandparents had little left in their savings. He spent 10 days in the hospital before he died. At his funeral, I recall a family friend saying it was a blessing he passed away so quickly, for otherwise the whole family might have been thrust into poverty. Can this happen again in America? Do people younger than I even realize how different things were just thirty-some years ago?

Even though we are in our early 50s and late 40s, my friends and I talk a lot about Medicare. We are all in the same boat, worried about elderly parents, our own futures and those of our kids. We share a concern that our elected representatives may be sacrificing the future in order to be reelected next time. None of us is willing to accept that. In fact, 1997 polls showed more than 60 percent of Americans want Congress to leave Medicare alone. That means more people support the Medicare social contract, enacted 33 years ago, than they do the so-called Contract With America that Congress tried to fulfill.

Having said all that, I believe there is indeed room for Medicare reform. But before we ask senior citizens to pay more for health care, the rates Medicare pays doctors and hospitals should be slashed. Even if American doctors received 25 percent less from Medicare, they would still be the richest M.D.'s in the world. And if hospitals received less money from Medicare, more of them might be forced to close their underutilized facilities.

I'm willing to pay more taxes to ensure that there will be a Medicare program for my parents, myself and my daughter. I am committed to the social contract this country entered into 33 years ago. And so are most of my friends and neighbors.

But I'm not sure Washington knows how we feel. That's why I'm worried about Medicare.

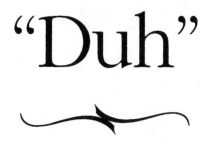

"Duh"

My 16-year-old daughter calls it a "duh." That's her genera-
tion's reaction to hearing the obvious. For example, when I
say to her, "If you don't get out of the house in five minutes,
you'll be late for school," she responds with, "Duh, Dad."

Now I'm no teenager, but I recently blurted out a "duh"
myself. It happened in early December 1997 when an advisory panel appointed by President Clinton and charged with
creating a Consumer Bill of Rights for Health Care issued its
report. This 34-member group, which deliberated for almost
a year, gave President Clinton a list of suggested consumer
safeguards aimed specifically at protecting the rights of people enrolled in health maintenance organizations and other
managed care plans—that's now most insured Americans.

Among the proposed rights: Consumers have the right
to obtain information on health plans, health professionals
and health care facilities. Also, consumers have the right to
a network of doctors and hospitals large enough to prevent
long waits for care. If consumers are seriously ill, they must
be granted direct access to specialists without having to wait
for permission. Also, consumers have the right to go to an
emergency room without getting permission from an insurer
first—if it seems like the reasonable thing to do.

Wait, there's more: Doctors have the right to tell consumers about treatment options that might not be covered
by a managed care plan. There's also a provision to protect
medical records and patient confidentiality.

President Clinton didn't even wait a day before announcing he'd ask Congress to put most of these recommended health care rights into law. "Duh," he implied, and I have to agree. Haven't we figured out by now that this country needs fundamental consumer protections to guard against the more powerful forces in health care doing as they please?

Well, I thought this sentiment was obvious and bipartisan, but apparently it's not. Upon hearing of the proposed bill of health care rights, Republican leaders and business leaders announced their opposition. Many said government shouldn't tell health plans what to do. Some employers cried that rights will raise health care costs. And with arguments such as these, the lines were quickly drawn. This could have been a "duh"—one of those rare moments when we take a break from lobbing buzzwords such as *big government* and make some progress. But don't count on any health care bill of rights sailing through Congress anytime soon.

As I sit here pondering all this, I wonder if our nation's founders had similar problems drafting the original Bill of Rights. Were costs a consideration when legislators proposed our right to free speech or to freedom of the press? What entity other than the government can protect a citizen's right to privacy?

What the president's panel recommended was a modest set of obvious protections every consumer in an HMO or managed care plan should have. There's no ulterior motive here. And if it weren't for a few powerful grinches, the whole proposal could be wrapped up like a wonderful gift for everyone—one that would take some of the worry out of getting sick!

Dinosaurs

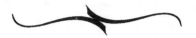

Twenty-seven years ago, a friend of mine was rushed to the hospital while suffering a heart attack. After he was stabilized in the emergency room, he was supposed to be shifted to the coronary care unit. But he couldn't be moved. It wasn't his condition that forced him to stay. No, the truth was that there were no beds available in the coronary unit. It was full. In fact, there were no beds available in the entire hospital. For five days, Richard remained in the emergency room until a bed opened up in another part of the facility.

That was 1971, and similar scenes were often being played out in most of America's hospitals. But if you walk into the average hospital today, you'll notice that more than half the beds are empty. In 1996, for the first time in this century, hospital occupancy fell below 50 percent. By the year 2000, more than 60 percent of the nation's hospital beds will be without patients.

This is a strange turn of events for institutions that for a long time were viewed as temples. In the early part of this century, most hospitals were built by religious groups to serve their parishioners and the community at large. In big cities, municipal governments erected large public hospitals for growing urban populations. And rural areas got small hospitals thanks to the ingenuity of physicians. In fact, most rural hospitals were owned by local physicians.

Hospitals cured the sick, fixed the broken and cared for the dying. Every community aspired to have its own hospital, if not several. A hospital was a sign of progress, a statement by the residents that they cared for one another.

As such, hospitals became the center of the community's health. They had the equipment, the personnel and the know-how to care for thousands of people each year. And for the most part, hospitals were the only place such services could be performed.

That is no longer the case. Over the last 15 years, new technologies have allowed practitioners to perform complex procedures in nonhospital settings safely and routinely. In fact, my family recently spent a New Year's Day with a friend who had her gallbladder removed just four days earlier. She never set foot in the hospital. The procedure was performed at an outpatient surgery center, bloodlessly, with a fiberscopic instrument called a laparoscope. She went home the same day. Experiences such as this are a big reason hospital occupancy rates have been declining since the early 1980s.

Despite this decline in occupancy, few hospitals (just several hundred out of more than 5,000) have closed since 1990. But there is no question that in the years to come, many more facilities will be gone. In fact, the "merger mania" now taking place in the hospital industry is merely an attempt by some hospitals to secure their own survival in the years ahead.

Hospital beds are empty because we don't need them. Since 1990, more surgeries are performed annually in outpatient settings than in hospitals. Medications are replacing many surgeries. And new equipment, such as the laparoscope, is making hospital stays obsolete.

Because hospitals have had such an historic and important role in our community and our lives, most people are disturbed by hospital closings. But the fact is that hospitals have become health care dinosaurs. In fact, the hospital industry is to the 1990s what the livery stable industry was to the 1890s—a hallowed but dying part of America. And just like livery stables, hospitals as we know them will be basically extinct in a matter of decades.

While some mourn the passing of hospitals, I, for one, do not. In fact, when I hear of a hospital closing, I think of it as progress. Every time one shuts down, we are saving money and shifting much-needed personnel to other community health services such as nursing homes and assisted living communities, where there is a shortage of well-trained workers.

In the past, a hospital—a single building—was the center of health in the community. But today, we are spreading our health care expertise throughout the entire community. That's better for everybody.

Outsmarting Mother Nature?

My great-grandmother died in Chicago in the late 1890s from what was then called childbirth fever. She was only 28 years old. Her death was not unusual in the nineteenth century—or in any century prior to this one. Women routinely died from infections that occurred during childbirth because the only treatments available for infection were compresses, prayers and luck.

All that changed with the development of antibiotics in the 1930s. Diseases and illnesses that had been almost sure death sentences were stopped in their tracks—including childbirth fever.

Antibiotics revolutionized medicine because they worked so well. Doctors even began prescribing antibiotic therapy to patients in order to prevent infections from occurring, especially in hospitals, which were natural breeding grounds for germs. Why risk it? the theory went. By the 1950s, antibiotics—especially penicillin—were the most prescribed medications in the United States. The medical world boasted that man had conquered nature.

That's turned out to not be so true. In fact, our dependency on antibiotics appears to be backfiring.

In the late 1970s, studies began to appear suggesting that many of the microbes that had been successfully wiped out by antibiotics for years were becoming resistant to them. Other studies showed that consumers were having to take larger doses of antibiotics for longer periods in order for them to be as effective. In other words, nature was fighting back.

Most in medicine, though, tried to dismiss these findings. Doctors presumed that new and more effective antibiotics would keep coming. Hadn't that been the case for almost 50 years? Maybe, but the possibility of finding a new antibiotic or wonder drug just in time—and having history repeat itself—grows dimmer by the day.

We know that, in part, because the hospital infection rate has been climbing for the last 20 years. Studies show that 10 percent of people who enter hospitals get infections they did not have when they were admitted. That's twice the percentage of just 15 years ago. And most sobering of all: According to the Centers for Disease Control and Prevention, 80,000 people a year die from hospital-acquired infections. That's an epidemic.

There's also new evidence that we have overused antibiotics so much that there are now some bacterial strains that are completely resistant to every antibiotic—even vancomycin, considered *the* most powerful antibiotic available. In a recent four-year period, the resistance to the drug vancomycin increased by nearly 700 percent.

Obviously, man has not overcome nature. We have abused a gift and are beginning to suffer the consequences. We are in a race that at this point has us in second place. As a society, we are finding out the hard way that we need to be more prudent and thoughtful in how we use, or abuse, any great scientific finding and development.

Now our focus has to be on preventing infections from spreading. You'll be shocked to know that the number one cause of hospital infections spreading from one patient to another is hospital staffers not washing their hands! And pneumonia, the most common hospital-acquired infection, can be largely prevented with an existing pneumonia vaccine. But doctors are not suggesting or giving the vaccine routinely, despite calls by the federal government for doctors to do so.

It's strange, though, how things have turned out. If antibiotics had been available in my great-grandmother's day, she and most women would have gotten through childbirth with ease. But 100 years from now, my great-granddaughter may be at the same risk as my great-grandmother was more than a century ago. That's scary!

The Party's Over!

I've been warning senior citizens to think carefully before joining a Medicare health maintenance organization. I have always been concerned that many of these health plans were luring seniors in with all sorts of extra benefits—benefits that might suddenly be cut if the HMOs found themselves losing money. I have also feared repercussions if the federal government decided not to be quite as generous with Medicare reimbursements as it has been.

Well, it seems the party's over. As part of 1997's balanced budget agreement, the federal government decided Medicare HMOs are going to have to live with reimbursement increases averaging only 2 percent, compared with an average of 9 percent in the previous few years. Also, a number of big insurers with Medicare managed care plans, such as Humana and Blue Cross/Blue Shield, are only now discovering how costly treating some seniors can be. The result?

In December 1997, a number of managed care plans announced they were either eliminating some of the extra benefits—items such as low-cost prescriptions, eyeglasses and hearing aids—or were requiring members to pay more for them. For example, a Blue Cross/Blue Shield Medicare HMO in Pennsylvania increased its 1998 monthly premiums by as much as $35 and dropped prescription drug coverage for some of its 21,000 members. A New Jersey Medicare plan did the same thing and also decided eye exams and dental coverage could no longer be offered. Name almost any state, and I'll show you a Medicare HMO that's beating a fast retreat from once-celebrated extra benefits.

I should note that none of these plans is going out of business. Nor are they dropping mandated coverage—that's against the law. At minimum, Medicare HMOs must provide the same services traditional Medicare provides (for example, regular mammograms). As for disgruntled seniors contemplating returning to traditional fee-for-service Medicare, that's an option riddled with new problems.

The major problem involves getting back supplemental, or Medigap, insurance once you've been in an HMO. It may not be simple. Medigap insurance is the extra private insurance most Medicare recipients carry to pay for whatever the federal program doesn't cover, such as prescriptions. Federal law requires insurers to issue a policy to anyone initially signing up for Medicare, regardless of his medical condition. But if a person drops the insurance, which most people who join Medicare HMOs do, the insurance company is not required to reissue the policy. And even if a policy is reissued, it does not have to be at the old rate. Many Medicare HMO members considering a switch back to fee-for-service insurance won't be able to afford this now more-expensive supplemental insurance and, therefore, will probably have to stay where they are.

And the problem is only going to get worse. Seventy percent of the nation's HMOs lost money in 1997. Most of them offer Medicare plans. To cut their losses, their only choice is to cut back on the extra benefits used to attract large numbers of seniors—a tactic that worked and is still working. After all, 100,000 seniors a month are enrolling in Medicare HMOs. As of January 1998, 16 percent of the Medicare-eligible population had signed up. That's almost 5 million people.

There's another question: How long will many of these insurance companies stay in the HMO business if they continue to lose money? I mean, I'd rather take my chances underwriting the risk of auto accidents than try to predict how much health care costs are going to rise!

And complicating it all are our nation's politicians. When President Clinton proposed his ill-fated health reform plan in 1993, many politicians on both sides of the aisle screamed to keep the government out of health care and let the market do its thing. To a large extent, those politicos won, and the market has taken its own course.

The trouble is that the course seems to be failing in many ways. If more than three-quarters of the HMOs are in poor financial straits, how sound is the market? And if consumers are losing benefits because of poor corporate management or bad federal policy, is the market working? The irony of it all is that now, as managed care companies are hurting and consumers are the ones screaming, politicians are threatening to take action against the HMOs. In other words, they want to regulate what they said shouldn't be regulated. Sadly, it's all a game. And we consumers are the pawns.

So what should a Medicare enrollee do? If you're in an HMO and like it, definitely stay in it, but don't count on the extra benefits to be there forever. And if you're thinking of leaving a plan to go back to the traditional Medicare program, shop around to see if you can once again get affordable Medigap coverage. If you're considering a Medicare HMO for the first time, look for a plan with plenty of doctors and hospitals to choose from and a reputation for high-quality care—just what the rest of Americans in the managed care marketplace must sort out.

In other words, my senior citizen friends, welcome to the club. There was a free lunch when the HMO wanted you to enroll, but the truth is that there is no free lunch in health care—especially for Medicare recipients.

School for Scandal

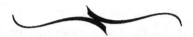

"Wash your hands with soap, Charles, or you'll go home hungry!"

I heard those words some 45 years ago, on my second day in kindergarten. It was afternoon snack time, and my teacher, Mrs. Major, had just marched some 20 of us boys down to the boys' bathroom. She threw open the door and led us right up to a line of sinks.

"Now listen carefully," she said in a tone of voice I would not hear again until I met my first drill sergeant. "Every day before we eat, I am going to bring you here to wash your hands. Dirty hands spread germs. And germs make us sick. I don't want sick children in my class. And your mothers and fathers don't want you sick, either."

Hand Washing 101, as I call it, was my very first public school health lesson, and it was far from my last. In first grade, we learned about polio. We saw filmstrips of kids in iron lungs. We were warned about using public swimming pools in the summer. And the next year, with the development of the polio vaccine, all of us became polio pioneers—kids given shots right in school. I think I still have my vaccination certificate in the same box that contains my old baseball cards.

Fast forward to the 1970s. School boards and state legislators decide that school-based public health classes are too costly. By the 1980s, preparing kids to compete in the new global economy becomes the priority.

So what's been the result? Well, according to a 1996 federal report, fewer than half of the nation's schools now require students to take even one health education course. And where health education is required, the only topics discussed in most cases are the dangers of alcohol and drug use, along with HIV prevention. Not unimportant areas for schools to focus upon. But it's not the same. It's no substitute for attending to children's overall health.

In most schools today, you can no longer find a public health nurse. Instead, there's someone on staff called a "school health aide." Only a handful of states insist that these folks have prior training.

And in the 1990s, when we finally have scientific proof that exercise is a key factor in maintaining a lifetime of good health, our kids are getting half the physical education time in school that they did 30 years ago. This, too, is due to local and state funding cutbacks.

So big deal, you say. What's the problem? Let parents teach their kids what Mrs. Major and the school nurse once taught. And why should we pay for school physical education when soccer fields are filled on weekends and inner-city basketball courts are crowded day and night?

Well, the problem is that things aren't quite what they appear. Though fitness seems popular, the truth is that American kids are the most obese children in the world. The average American teenager is physically weaker than his father or mother was 40 years ago.

In addition, almost half of the children coming to their first day of school have not received their vaccinations.

Despite all our progress, diseases we thought were on the wane, such as tuberculosis and whooping cough, are on the rise again.

Isn't it funny that some of our politicians might have us believe that it's OK to cut school health and physical education programs because they don't directly relate to job skills and the learning that kids need for the twenty-first century? Gosh, I'm worried that our kids may be too sick and feeble to enjoy the good times that are supposedly coming.

Over
the
Counter

Have you ever wondered why birth control pills are still available only by prescription? After all, most brands have been on the market for more than 35 years. More women—about a billion—use the Pill than use any other prescription medication. So why can't it be bought over the counter?

Here's another question: How come so many drugs available over the counter in foreign countries are still sold only by prescription in the United States?

If this were a quiz, your answer to both questions would be "safety." And in theory, you'd be right. But there are many products sold only by prescription that have been shown to be as safe as similar products sold over the counter. So what's going on?

We all know drugs—even legal ones—can be dangerous. Because of that, we have an elaborate system of federal control over the entire pharmaceutical industry. No product—prescription or over the counter—can come on the market unless it meets certain standards. For the most part, the system works pretty well.

In the 1800s, controls didn't exist. Anybody could make anything, label it a medicine and sell it to an unsuspecting public. But products became more sophisticated. So did the clamor for better consumer protection. Soon after the turn of the century, the forerunner to our current U.S. Food and Drug Administration was created.

Since then, no single aspect of the health care system has had more of an impact on consumer health and longevity than pharmaceutical products. From sulfa drugs to antibiotics, we live longer and better because of the ever-growing list of new and important medications. And the twenty-first century looks even brighter.

But as we get closer to the year 2000, we must also recognize that we have become better medical consumers. We are more knowledgeable about drugs and medical services than ever. Studies show that consumers use over-the-counter products responsibly and effectively, meaning we know how to use many medications without ever consulting a physician.

The government has begun to recognize this by making many more formerly prescription-only drugs available over the counter. Many of the antihistamines and heartburn medications on drugstore shelves were behind the pharmacy counter just a few years ago. In February 1996, the FDA approved the hair-restoring product Rogaine for over-the-counter status. But none of these products got there without a fight. And that brings me back to the question of birth control pills.

More studies have been done on birth control pills than on any other pharmaceutical product in history. The conclusion: They're safe and effective. So why require a prescription?

Doctors!

Physicians have lobbied against changing the Pill's status because they say if it's available over the counter, women will stop coming in for gynecological examinations. Yet studies show that doctors write most birth control prescriptions when patients aren't present. It's not the women they're worried about as much as making sure that they—as doctors—are indispensable.

And that's the way it is with many products that remain behind the counter. For example, in 1995, the Food and Drug Administration refused to allow the antiviral drug acyclovir, extremely effective in treating herpes, to be sold without a prescription. Even though medical studies show acyclovir is quite safe and a panel of experts recommended it for over-the-counter status, physicians opposed this. And today, it is still a prescription-only medication. So now fewer people get the drug than might, and the herpes epidemic is growing.

It is time to change the system so that prescription products that have been safely on the market for many years may be granted over-the-counter status. While it is essential that we be protected from toxic and dangerous products, it is also important to remember that medications are made to heal, not to protect anyone's medical turf.

Obsolete?

I upset my family doctor a while ago. I went to see him because I was sure I was suffering from a sinus infection and all my home remedies had failed. I needed an antibiotic.

At my appointment, the nurse weighed me and took my blood pressure, and then the doctor entered the examining room. He asked about my symptoms, tapped my sinuses, looked in my ears and listened to my chest. He confirmed my diagnosis—sinus infection. He handed me a prescription for an antibiotic, along with a bill for $45. He shook my hand and was headed for the door when I stopped him in his tracks.

"You know," I said, "I think most family doctors and other primary care physicians are obsolete."

He turned around in surprise.

"In fact," I went on, "even many procedures *specialists* perform could be done by trained technicians. Since every other business in the world seems to be reengineering, I think it's time doctoring be reengineered, too. We could probably cut the number of doctors in the United States from 600,000 to 400,000 without any ill effect on health care!"

He sat down. He looked stunned.

"What do you mean?" he asked, obviously irritated. "Doctors are better trained than ever before. Today, we have the knowledge and technology to diagnose and treat conditions that were virtually untreatable as recently as 50 years ago. It wasn't that long ago that virtually nothing could be done about cancer or heart disease or most other serious problems."

"But that's exactly my point," I argued. "The real progress

---

made in medicine has not been due to the improved skill of doctors, but to technological advances. We treat cancer with chemotherapy, radiation and surgery. People with heart disease are given a pill, a pacemaker or some other mechanical device. We replace worn-out or broken joints with artificial ones. None of this requires a doctor. A well-trained nurse or technician could perform most of these procedures."

He remained silent, but I was on a roll!

"Even diagnosis is technology-driven," I continued. "Unless the problem is an obvious one, such as my sinus infection, you send the patient for lab tests or x-rays. Why? Because those results are more reliable than even your best educated guess."

"But what about surgery?" he countered. "Don't you need a skilled physician to do complicated brain surgery or a coronary bypass procedure?"

"In my opinion," I suggested, "today's surgeon is basically a technician."

"Look," I said, "I'm not suggesting that we get rid of doctors. Quite the opposite. We need to put doctors to better use. Considering the time and cost of your medical education, it seems ridiculous for you to be tapping my sinuses, looking in my ears and listening to my chest. A nurse practitioner could do that. She's well trained and has excellent skills, and studies show nurse practitioners could handle 90 percent of all primary care. You should be doing more advanced work, such as complicated transplants or working with rare conditions. In other words, you're overtrained for what you do!"

He got up. There were other patients waiting. We shook hands again, but this time he moved to the door more slowly. As he left, he looked back at me and said, "I never thought of it that way. Maybe you're right."

Of Little Importance

When I was growing up in Chicago in the 1950s, we never went to a drugstore to fill a prescription. In sleet or snow, rain or shine, our neighborhood druggist always delivered to our home. The delivery arrived quickly, sometimes in less than 30 minutes. And there was no paperwork. Our family doctor called the pharmacist directly. My mother could also order a refill over the phone.

These memories came back to me a few years ago, when the Rite Aid and Revco drugstore chains announced that they were going to merge. Now the deal never happened, but later Revco did sell out to another drugstore giant, CVS. But what struck me as strange at the time—and still does today as chain after chain combines—is the importance the combining companies attach to the deals when they present them to the public.

For example, in announcing the Rite Aid-Revco union, the companies claimed that the merger would make the new entity more competitive while better serving consumers. And they were frank in saying that their survival rested on commanding a greater share of the marketplace.

For a few days after the announcement, a great debate was held in the media about drugstore mergers. Critics spoke of the final demise of the already dwindling neighborhood pharmacy. Advocates contended that drugstore mergers would mean greater efficiency and lower costs.

Actually, both sides were right. But both sides were missing the real point. Pharmacies, whether large national chains or independently owned drugstores, are obsolete. And they have been for at least a decade. It's time we face that fact and start looking at newer, cheaper and more consumer friendly ways to get medications into people's hands.

Forty years ago, the local pharmacist was an essential part of the community. For most prescriptions, she had to mix or grind up pill ingredients on site. But over the last three decades, that has changed. Today, the pharmacist in the store you visit mostly transfers pills and capsules from a large jar to a smaller one. No one needs five years of training at a pharmacy college to learn how to do that.

Some pharmacists quarrel with me about their role. While they concede that they no longer do as much mixing, mashing and melding as they used to, they insist that they play an important role in passing along information to the consumer. But even that is overstated. Most pharmacists, whether at a family-owned store or a Wal-Mart, don't spend much time talking with customers about their prescriptions. They hand out computer-generated printouts.

There are better ways to get prescription drugs. One is by mail order, which is already a successful and growing method of pharmaceutical distribution. It is the perfect way to deliver needed medications to people who are unable to leave their homes or who live in rural or isolated areas. Plus, it is the ideal way to refill prescriptions or purchase them in bulk. And the same printed information can be inserted into the package.

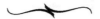

But why stop there? There is no reason that you should not be able to fill a prescription 24 hours a day at a terminal similar to your bank's automatic teller machine. Your doctor could enter your prescription on a smart card, and you could obtain your pills or potions anywhere in the country your card is accepted.

And we can even go back to the days of drugstore delivery. If Domino's and Pizza Hut can take an order, make a pizza, cook it and deliver it in less than 30 minutes for more than half the people in the country, why can't we do the same with medications? We can. The same innovative, entrepreneurial thinking will, I believe, make it commonplace.

All these big drugstore chain mergers are similar to the railroad mergers of the 1950s. They sound big and important, but they're really just a sign of the end of an era.

They All Look Alike to Me

In 1996, two hospitals in Pennsylvania were stripped of their tax-exempt, charitable status. In the case of Harrisburg Hospital in Pennsylvania, the judge took action because the company that owned the institution used hospital revenues to buy physician practices, medical office buildings, clinics and a medical equipment business—all with the intention of making money.

The case is being appealed, but what happened to Harrisburg Hospital is not unique. All across the country what we've thought of as charitable hospitals—usually affiliated with religious groups or universities—are losing tax-exempt status. Local courts and officials are deciding there's not much basis anymore to treat such facilities differently than their for-profit competitors. And they're right!

All hospitals today face similar challenges and pressures. There are too many empty beds, and insurers (including the government) insist on paying a lot less for care. So if a hospital is going to survive—and some have already closed—it has to figure out new and ingenious ways to attract patients and corner the market. And that's where many not-for-profit, or charitable, institutions have crossed the "charity" line. They've purchased physician practices, created new for-profit businesses on the side and paid administrators six-figure salaries, letting everyone in the community know that they aren't the same institutions that the people's Sunday offerings helped to build. And to top it all off, many of these facilities are merging with former competitors or even selling out to for-profit hospital chains such as Columbia/HCA or Humana.

At the community level, there's great controversy over the arrival of for-profit hospitals. Critics claim that for-profits cut quality, replace skilled nurses with less qualified personnel and put shareholder interests ahead of patient care. Proponents argue that for-profits often breathe new life into what was a dying local hospital, manage medical care more efficiently and provide a windfall of tax dollars to communities fighting to keep their budgets balanced.

So who's right? Let's take a look at quality of care. Ten years ago, for-profit hospitals were accused of performing excessive numbers of unnecessary tests and surgeries, keeping people in the hospital too long and charging too much for their services. But that's not the case anymore. In fact, some studies suggest today's for-profit hospital may be more medically and economically efficient than its not-for-profit competitor. And since when did we become critical of profit making in medical care? Doctors have been interested in making money for years!

And what about the tax issue? Recent court cases suggest that most tax-exempt hospitals can't adequately explain the charitable services they supposedly provide. I once heard a hospital administrator tell a judge that the directional signal the hospital installed on the road in front of his facility was a charitable contribution to the community. The judge laughed as hard as I did.

Remember: Charitable hospitals came about because private, physician-owned hospitals wouldn't serve the poor. Today, many of our so-called charitable facilities have closed their emergency rooms and turned away the uninsured.

Now I'm not saying there aren't any hospitals around anymore that are committed to their communities. But if there was any doubt before, health really is a business today. It's time we do away with tax exemption for hospitals and tax them all! Local taxing authorities would then receive a portion of any hospital's financial windfall, and the community could decide how to use the funds to provide other needed services.

What
to Eat

✦

Mrs. Swan was my fourth grade teacher back in 1956. One morning when we got to school, she attached a large poster to the blackboard. It pictured a pyramid divided into sections. Inside each section were drawings of fruits and vegetables, meats, a carton of milk and assorted other foods.

"What's that?" my friend Ned asked.

"I don't know," I said. "We're probably going to learn about Egypt."

"You guys are so stupid," Joe, the class know-it-all, boomed. "Don't you know cave drawings when you see them? All those drawings were made by cavemen and represent the world around them."

Before I had a chance to tell Joe that cavemen didn't have milk cartons, Mrs. Swan called the class to order.

As we later learned, the poster represented a food guide pyramid similar to the one that is now put out by the U.S. Department of Agriculture. It shows the consensus of nutritional experts on what types of foods are healthiest for most people and the percentage of our daily diets that should come from each group.

At the time Mrs. Swan was teaching about nutrition, there was very little controversy surrounding the recommendations. There was the meat group, the milk group, the breads and cereals group and the fruits and vegetables group, all of which she had arranged in a pyramidal form. In case you've forgotten, foods at the bottom of the food pyramid are considered the most healthy, and you're encouraged to eat them. Foods up at the top you can also eat, but sparingly.

In Mrs. Swan's class, I remember thinking how lucky my friends and I were to be alive. Unlike ever before, our scientific knowledge was giving us undisputable answers to questions previous generations only guessed at. Little did I know that the next few decades would feature a battle over what truly belongs at the bottom of the pyramid.

New studies in the 1970s began to shed light on the dangers of cholesterol. So some nutritionists lobbied the government to promote low-cholesterol eating. Their lobbying was successful, and the next guidelines also included a group for fats, sweets and alcohol, which were to be eaten rarely.

In the mid-1980s, the food pyramid as we know it, with six food groups, was developed. But during the 1990s, even more controversy emerged. By comparing the diet of Americans with that of people in other countries and comparing the frequency of specific diseases, nutrition experts concluded the food pyramid was all wrong and again clamored for adjustments. Some groups devised whole new pyramids, such as the Mediterranean and Asian pyramids, based on their interpretation of the data. But the data keep changing, which is making it increasingly difficult for the official pyramid creators to know which end is up.

For example, consider the highly publicized study of the mid-1990s that reviewed previous findings linking fat intake to breast cancer. For 10 years, medical researchers had been arguing that the reason Chinese women have lower breast cancer rates than American women is because their diets are lower in fat. This so-called finding has been used in convincing American women to lower their fat intakes, and it has had a great deal to do with the USDA's placement of fat at the very top of the pyramid. But now evidence suggests there may not be as strong a connection between fat intake and breast cancer. So should the food pyramid be changed again? To be honest, I don't know.

I've learned a lot since my introduction to food guides 40 years ago. First, the food pyramid is simply a guide based on the best knowledge at the time. If you don't like what you see, rest assured—it will change in very short order.

On the one hand, the food pyramid carries a great deal of clout. Dietitians use it for school lunch planning. Nutritionists use it to teach proper menu planning. And the fact that food industry and health interest groups lobby so hard over where certain food groups are placed in it signifies its impact.

On the other hand, perhaps the problem with the food pyramid is that it's a pyramid at all. A better symbol might be building blocks that can be rearranged from time to time without everything toppling down. In fact, those blocks may make it even easier for consumers to understand what's best for them and at the same time take some of the politics out of what we eat.

After
Work

My late father-in-law retired at age 53 after 30 years with the same employer. During his first 12 years of retirement, his former employer paid for all his health care. Every penny of it. They even paid all of my mother-in-law's expenses. When he turned 65, he enrolled in Medicare, but his former employer continued to pay for those health care costs not covered by the program. My father-in-law died in 1991. We figured out that his former employer had paid for his medical costs for close to 70 years, about half of them as a retiree.

Several years ago, a U.S. Circuit Court of Appeals ordered General Motors to provide free health care benefits to 50,000 workers who retired early between 1974 and 1988. The court said, "The company had improperly reneged on a promise to pay for health care for those employees and their spouses for life."

Retiree medical costs are rising for American businesses, so it's not surprising that GM tried to wiggle out of this agreement. It didn't succeed, but the fact that it even tried should make us all sit up and take notice and get used to a leaner, meaner future.

That's going to be tough. As recently as 20 years ago, large companies didn't think twice about offering lifelong benefits to employees. Health care coverage was one of those benefits. And why not? Health care was cheap, and health insurance premiums were low, in part because after World War II, the workforce was young and healthy. On the other hand, life expectancy was short. In 1970, a male worker who retired at 65 lived only five years more. Today, that same worker lives at least 15 years more.

Also in the 1950s and 1960s, the economy was booming, and manufacturing jobs were increasing, so companies needed to attract and keep more workers. The cheapest, most effective way to do that was to promise benefits far into the future. By the mid-1960s, more than three-quarters of America's largest corporations promised and paid their workers full health care benefits after retirement.

But as the General Motors case clearly shows us, big businesses see things quite differently now. Health care costs have soared since the 1960s, and companies can no longer afford generous plans for their active workers, much less for their former workers. In fact, according to a government report, less than half of America's largest employers are now providing health benefits for former employees. And there are no laws that require companies to provide health care benefits to any employee, much less to retirees.

I'm not here to lambast big business for this. Frankly, I think it's unrealistic for an employer to pay for the health care of a retiree for 34 years—as was the case with my father-in-law's employer. It just doesn't make economic sense.

But what does? We can't ignore the fact that 60 million baby boomers will soon reach retirement age. What will happen if they retire before they're eligible for Medicare? Will they be able to afford high-priced health premiums? Evidence already suggests that they can't. Most of America's newly uninsured are people in their 50s who retired, or were forced to retire, without health benefits.

This is disturbing news. And while we all search for answers, I suggest that those of us under age 65 start planning now. If you anticipate early retirement, start checking out health insurance options such as traditional individual indemnity, or fee-for-service, policies or managed care plans. Under the latter, you usually get more coverage for your money than with an indemnity plan. And even if you retire at 65 when you're eligible for Medicare, it might be wise to consider a Medicare health maintenance organization. That way you won't need to carry supplemental Medicare insurance, which has been skyrocketing in price the last few years.

When my father-in-law retired back in 1957, he knew he didn't have to worry about health care costs for the rest of his life. Things are a lot different for his son-in-law. I'll be worrying about them until the day I die.

PART V

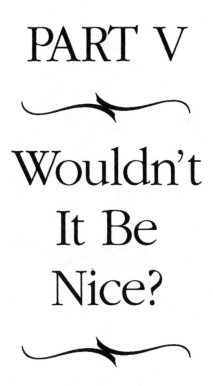

Wouldn't
It Be
Nice?

Sure, I've talked about what's wrong. But I hope you've sensed my strong feelings of optimism about the future of medicine, the advancement of medical consumerism and the potential for more people to live longer, healthier and more productive lives. I hope, too, that I have been able to energize your optimism, as well. What's wrong with today's health care system is the lack of consumer focus. The more empowered, involved and demanding we are of the system, the better it will be.

So I end this book with examples of how it can be. But these are not just pipe dreams because the things I talk about in the ensuing pages are already happening. They are harbingers of a bright future. And that's truly exciting.

The Way
It
Should Be

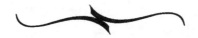

Not long ago, I received a phone call from a Wisconsin resident who was amazed at the treatment he's been getting from his health maintenance organization. "You won't believe it," he said. "For the past three weeks, this nurse has been regularly checking up on me. She calls to see if I'm taking my medication, if it's causing any problems and if I am getting better. She has even offered to send someone out to my house if I'm having trouble following my doctor's orders. Boy, business must be bad at the HMO if they can spend that much time on me."

Actually, just the opposite is true. What this man's HMO is doing is something called disease management. It's the latest trend in managed care and, in my opinion, one of the best. If done right, disease management benefits both the consumer and the HMO.

Disease management programs are designed to keep a consumer in close contact with a medical team once the patient leaves the doctor's office. This is an especially good way to monitor people with chronic conditions such as asthma, diabetes or hypertension since the health of these people may vary day to day and because taking medicine "as directed" can make a big difference with chronic conditions.

The assigned team may include a specialist, a pharmacist employed or retained by the HMO and a nurse who also specializes in the condition. And in a curious twist to today's managed care environment, patients with chronic conditions who belong to an HMO with a disease management program are actually encouraged to visit the HMO often. Here again, the idea is that the more regular one's contact is with a medical team, the more likely it is that health problems will not flare up. That, of course, is great for the health of the patient and for the financial strength of the managed care company.

Are disease management programs working? It sure seems like it. One study conducted at PCS Health Systems found that a group of employees with diabetes enrolled in one HMO cut their lost workdays by 63 percent. There was a 72 percent drop in hospital stays and a 71 percent reduction in emergency room visits. Plus, there was a direct medical cost savings of more than $1,200 per year, per patient. All thanks to disease management.

Disease management is not without controversy, however. The biggest question has to do with the roles drug companies play. Right now, some of the big pharmaceutical giants contract with HMOs to provide the services. Critics contend that drug companies shouldn't have such a direct role in patient care and have a built-in conflict of interest— such as pushing their own products. There's also some concern that drug companies are far more interested in learning how their prescription is doing financially compared with other remedies on the market than they are in patient health.

Plus, some people worry that an HMO's or a drug company's corporate profits could lead to compromises on patient care, especially if profits begin to decline. Will follow-up become less frequent? Will less expensive, possibly less effective drugs be used? These are all legitimate issues that need to be watched.

But so far, disease management programs have proved to be winners for both consumers and managed care companies. And why not? This is the way medicine should have always been delivered. Sadly, that has not been the case. And it's still the case for most people.

It's ludicrous to think that a single professional, namely a physician, has all the knowledge, resources and time to spend on every patient that crosses her portal. That's especially true in a world in which just about every health care professional has special training that sets her apart from other medical colleagues. Who knows more than a pharmacist about the effects and side effects of a drug? Nurses are specially trained to work with individual consumers when it comes to health education and treatment follow-up. There are many special health care technicians, such as those who fit people with prosthetic devices, who bring a wealth of training and knowledge to a health care problem. But unless a consumer is enrolled in a managed care plan that offers a disease management program, coordination between all these entities just doesn't happen.

That's why the man from Wisconsin was so surprised that his HMO was so interested in following up on his problem. In his entire life, he had never encountered as much attention from health care professionals.

Disease management is going to be the reason managed

care succeeds. No matter what happens to individual managed care companies, the concept of disease management has already shown exactly how health care should be delivered.

Disease management programs are also going to move way beyond the most common conditions. As they grow, we'll begin to see programs helping people who suffer from Alzheimer's disease, incontinence or cancer. The idea is to bring a team approach to care for an individual. And interestingly, physicians may be the least involved professionals on a day-to-day basis.

Indeed, this has been a long time in coming. Up to now, most of us had to coordinate our own health services. If you needed a visiting nurse, you had to arrange it. When you needed a new prescription or were having problems with the one you were taking, the onus was on you to find the help and assistance you needed. Despite all the professional resources out there, the proverbial left hand rarely spoke to the right hand. As a result, many people suffered.

Frankly, it's too late to turn back now. Consumers who have used disease management programs like them. And consumer demand is what is now driving our health care system. In the years to come, these programs are going to become the norm in medical care delivery. And as a result, all of us will have better health care and better lives.

Prescribing Disclosure

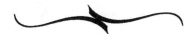

A 1995 U.S. Food and Drug Administration proposal, which is expected to be fully implemented by 2006, demonstrates how powerful the voice of the medical consumer has become.

In August 1995, the FDA proposed a program that would give consumers written information about the prescription medications they take. According to the plan, each time a consumer receives a drug from a pharmacy, he also receives a leaflet that clearly explains the approved uses of the drug, when it should not be used and any serious adverse reactions. The consumer is also told how to take the medication properly and warned of any cautions related to its use.

Under the plan, each leaflet looks the same—in other words, the format is standardized. That way there can be no variation from one pharmacy to another. Everyone is given the same information.

The program went into effect in 1996, with 75 percent compliance expected by the year 2000 and 95 percent by 2006.

This program, when it was announced, was great news for my friend Peggy. She refused to take any prescription medication because of three incidents she had with three different drugs. In each case, she had taken the prescription and suffered severe side effects—reactions so bad that she lost workdays and income. She had been given no warnings about possible side effects by either her doctor or her pharmacist. And Peggy was not alone in her refusal to take prescription medication. In fact, pharmaceutical industry studies suggest that close to half of all prescription medication dispensed is never taken.

While Peggy was happy, Ellen only grieved more. You see, her 72-year-old mother had been given a prescription by a doctor about four months before the FDA plan became public. Within a day, she unexpectedly died. It was later discovered by the local medical examiner, after Ellen fought for an investigation, that her mother's physician prescribed an inappropriate drug for her condition. He had not bothered to look at the warnings associated with the product. And Ellen's mother was given no information, written or verbal, that might have clued her in to the warnings.

This was not the first time the FDA proposed full disclosure on prescription medications, although it was the first time it was implemented. In the late 1970s, a similar program was put forth, only to be shot down by the drug industry and physicians. These groups used their money and political clout to keep consumers in the dark, arguing that the average citizen was not smart enough to understand the warnings. They told the FDA, Congress and, later, President Reagan that people would stop taking their medications if they knew all of the potential side effects.

They won then, but time has proven them wrong. The same studies that show half of all prescribed drugs are never used also show that a significant portion are not taken because consumers have too little information about proper use and side effects.

Over the last 15 years, medical and health consumerism has become a strong and growing force in America. It was consumers who demanded and won the uniform and informative food-labeling requirements that went into effect in 1994. Consumers are demanding to know the outcome rates of procedures performed in hospitals and by doctors. Those demands have won responses in more than a dozen states.

And now the consumer voice is being heard on prescription medication disclosure. Believe me, the FDA is not implementing this program because the pharmaceutical industry made demands. It's happening because of consumer demand. Consumers are finally being viewed both as customers and as a force to reckoned with. While it used to be that all matters medical had to get the beneficent nod of the medical community before government policy makers would act, today the tables have been turned. The consumer has become the top priority—something that should have been the case for years.

And this Food and Drug Administration prescription disclosure program is the biggest victory yet in the medical consumer's fight for useful information. And it is only the beginning of a new and growing consumer awareness of our power in the medical marketplace.

Helping Ourselves

All across America, there's a quiet health care revolution going on. No, it's not managed care. In fact, it has nothing to do with health insurance. And it doesn't involve a new medication or even an alternative therapy.

No, the revolution I'm talking about is so dynamic that more than 25 million people are involved. Some of them on a daily basis. And if it received better publicity, that number would probably double.

It's called the self-help movement, a mushrooming of groups comprised of laypeople who get together to learn more about a shared medical condition and how to deal with it.

It's estimated that there are 600,000 self-help groups throughout the country, and there is literally a group for every health condition. Membership is usually free. Lowell Levin, professor of public health at Yale University, calls the self-help movement "the quiet revolution." He and other experts who have studied self-help groups note that they provide to their members not only support but also vital information about effective treatments. They also serve as a viable way for consumers to swap information about practitioners and facilities that treat their malady.

My wife belongs to a self-help group for people with fibromyalgia. Fibromyalgia is a condition characterized by severe muscle pain that often makes the person suffering from it immobile. For a professional musician like my wife, the pain could be career ending. After years of seeing doctors, many of whom knew nothing about or weren't familiar with the condition, she was frustrated. Almost nothing they offered helped. Finally, my wife discovered a fibromyalgia self-help group in our community. At her first meeting, she was shocked to see more than 200 people in the room. Within an hour, she had connected with several other women who shared information about specific exercises and medications that had worked for them. In subsequent months and meetings, my wife learned more, and today, her fibromyalgia is under control and manageable.

Self-help is not a substitute for sound medical care or advice. But it's become a crucial addition to the traditional medical world. Think of it as taking a trip to a foreign land. You use a travel agency and read the guidebooks, but often the best information you get is from friends who have recently been there. Well, self-help in health matters is the same thing—advice and information from those who have medically been there.

Many medical professionals have latched onto self-help. Doctors and hospitals are beginning to refer their patients to local self-help groups to help them cope or deal with their conditions. Some doctors have also started attending self-help meetings in their specialities just to learn what patients say works. This underscores the power many of these groups have attained in their local communities. It also suggests that some of the ego of the medical world is being eroded. And that's important.

While medical specialists certainly know their fields,

they do not know everything. Their knowledge is limited by their patient pool, their continuing education and their ability to interact with colleagues throughout the country. Keeping up is not easy. New medications and treatment techniques come along rapidly. In fact, Yale's Levin suggests, with a wry wit, that the half-life of a medical fact is just five years.

But physicians also get little in the way of organized feedback from their patients. And often, patients do not tell doctors some of the things they've tried that the doctor did not know about. This has been seen quite clearly in the treatment of AIDS, in which many HIV positive people have used numerous treatment modalities without ever consulting their doctors. And self-help groups have been one of the ways that word of these nonphysician-controlled treatments has spread.

Even the experts are surprised at the scope of the self-help movement. A study published in 1997 in the journal *Social Policy* revealed that 25 million people participate in self-help. Up until then, the best guesses were that only about 10 million Americans were involved in such groups. But this new study—the first legitimate survey of the public on the subject—revealed astonishing results. Clearly, consumers are desperate for information that will help them treat and cope with their conditions.

Finding a self-help group in your area involves some research. First, ask your doctor or a nurse if either knows of a group appropriate for you. Or ask people you know who suffer from the same medical condition. Some state health departments keep lists of self-help organizations, and many national organizations, such as the Alzheimer's Association, maintain lists of local groups. There is even a nonprofit self-help clearinghouse you can call for help. It can be reached at 973-625-9565 or 800-FOR-MASH (in New Jersey) from 9:00 A.M. to 5:00 P.M. Eastern time on weekdays.

Self-help is like swapping advice over the backyard fence with a neighbor. It doesn't cost anything, it's usually quite friendly, and it's not intimidating. That's why people are joining in record numbers.

Seeing More Clearly

"It's amazing!"

Those were my father's exact words the day after he had a cataract removed from his left eye. The surgery was painless and stitchless. In fact, it lasted less than five minutes. And the next morning, when he went back to have the patch removed from his eye, the doctor handed him a newspaper and asked him to read it. The words were clearer than they had been in years, even the small print. He decided then and there that he would have his other eye fixed. And my mother decided to have her cataracts removed, as well.

My parents didn't belong to a Medicare health maintenance organization when they underwent the procedure. If they had, it is likely they would still be living with their old glasses and lousy vision. That's because, according to a study published in a June 1997 issue of the *Journal of the American Medical Association,* members of Medicare HMOs are half as likely to have cataract surgery than are Medicare beneficiaries in the regular fee-for-service system.

Now before you say "I told you so" about those cutthroat,

cost-containing HMOs, the researchers who did the study urge some caution on what conclusion to draw. On the one hand, seniors who belong to Medicare HMOs might be getting short-changed by managed care companies trying to eke out profits at the expense of patients' health. On the other hand, it's possible too many unnecessary cataract extractions are being performed under traditional fee-for-service Medicare.

Cataract surgery is one of the most common and effective surgical procedures Medicare recipients receive. Medicare pays more for cataract removals than for any other procedure—some $3.4 billion a year. Before Medicare HMOs became common, the government often criticized doctors for doing the operation unnecessarily or prematurely, suggesting that profit rather than medical need was the doctors' motive.

Medicare HMOs, on the other hand, can't "cash in" on cataract surgery in the same way since the HMOs receive a set monthly payment from the government for each enrollee regardless of that person's medical need. Plus, unlike the fee-for-service system, HMOs require a lot more approvals before anyone gets to have surgery. So it's not surprising to see some difference in the number of cataract surgeries performed on the population enrolled in Medicare HMOs. But a 50 percent difference? That really surprised researchers.

Could it be that fully half the cataract operations performed under the traditional Medicare reimbursement rules are unnecessary? Or conversely, are members of Medicare HMOs being denied something that has proven to be truly beneficial?

Well, I hate to disappoint critics of HMOs, but it's really not clear yet. This is the first study that's compared the likelihood of an operation being performed in an HMO versus a traditional insurance model. More studies are needed on some other commonly performed operations such as hysterectomies and coronary bypass surgeries. What we're left with in the meantime are several questions. Is managed care going to cut back on the number of all kinds of necessary surgeries performed? Are we beginning to see the extent to which patient care can be compromised at an HMO—especially if the care is expensive? It's this latter possibility that disturbs me—especially when I think about my parents' cataract surgeries and what a difference having clear vision has made to their lives and could make to the lives of millions of elderly Americans—many of whom are now being encouraged to join Medicare HMOs.

What this really points out is how we are changing the way we deliver health care without knowing if these changes are effective. There's no question that cataract surgery helps people. And there's also no doubt that modern technology has made the procedure as painless as a flu shot. It was not that many years ago that cataract patients were hospitalized (and immobilized) for up to two weeks. But in our drive to save money, are we sacrificing the quality of people's lives? In other words, is managed care taking a useful, relatively cheap medical procedure and rationing it simply to save a few dollars? Ultimately, won't those people who might qualify for the procedure still need it next month or next year? Sure, they will. But in the interim, their lives are limited because an insurance company, or the federal government, wants to save a few bucks.

I'm sorry—that's just not acceptable.

Consumers are already starting to stand up to HMOs and other managed care plans that deny them care their doctor deems necessary. It's evident in the number of appeals consumers are filing with their HMOs about denied services. The federal government reports that the number of appeals has been rising annually since 1990. This is only going to continue and grow. What this represents is consumers taking charge of the health care system. It's our health that's at stake here. It's also our money that's paying the bills. Where do insurers and legislators get off telling us what we can or cannot buy?

Health insurance in America was actually started by groups of doctors who created insurance companies in order to guarantee payment for services. Unfortunately, they never paid much attention to their customers. Instead of asking a customer what she needed, the insurer decided what it would provide. And since the insurer was really the physician, coverage became what the doctor decided was appropriate. So for more than 60 years, health care consumers had expensive and exotic treatments covered by insurance but were denied coverage for important services such as well-baby visits and mammograms.

But now the door has been opened to consumer control over the system. Unlike in the past, insurance companies, through HMOs and other managed care plans, must focus their sights on consumer satisfaction. Doctors are secondary in this new scheme of things. Unless customers are satisfied, health maintenance organizations can lose huge numbers of enrollees in a single swoop.

For example, if 5,000 employees of one company were enrolled with a single HMO—not an unusual occurrence these days—dissatisfaction by some of those employees could force the employer to change plans. In one day, a major exodus could occur. And managed care plans know that. That's why consumer satisfaction is so important.

That doesn't mean we will control insurance companies or determine what is medically necessary. Rather, it means the health care and health insurance industries will be responding with services and coverage levels that we want. Actually, it's simple business. We're the customers— they're the providers. If they cannot deliver what we want as customers, we'll take our business someplace else.

And these days, there's hardly a doctor, hospital or health insurance company that can afford to lose the business. In other words, even without internal surgery, the health industry is beginning to see more clearly.

A Dose
of Reality

Well, I'm happy.

As you've probably heard, the U.S. Food and Drug Administration has approved new rules for prescription drug advertising on television. Now, for the first time, these ads can tell you something about the medication. Up to now, all a commercial could do was advertise a product's name. Nothing more!

The old restrictions made for some pretty silly ads. I liked the one that showed close-ups of middle-aged people with smiling faces. After about 30 seconds, a product name came on the screen with the manufacturer's 800 number—which you could call for a brochure—followed by the announcer's last line, "Ask your doctor about Retin-A." Unless you knew Retin-A was an antiwrinkle product, you might have thought the ad was for a tooth whitener or even contact lenses.

Now, under the new FDA rules, manufacturers can say what the product is and make claims about its effectiveness. All the drug company has to do is be sure to mention any significant risks and provide a toll-free number or Internet address for more information. And all TV ads must be approved by the FDA to protect viewers from false or exaggerated statements.

I like the new rules for two major reasons. First, the more consumers know about prescription drugs, the more empowered they'll be. And consumer questions to physicians about drugs advertised on television force doctors to become better educated about medications. This can only enhance consumer-physician communication.

The second reason I like the new rules also has to do with consumer empowerment. For years, drug companies have directed all their advertising and marketing at physicians—ignoring us consumers, even though we often pay the prescription bills. As a result, medical organizations that publish journals and other publications—also aimed at doctors—have gotten rich from prescription ads. In 1996 alone, the American Medical Association took in 40 percent more in ad revenues, mostly from their publications, than the year before—a whopping $54 million. The AMA boasted in their own publications that total revenues, from all sources, were the highest in history.

We all know the AMA is a very powerful lobby for doctors. Despite representing only about half of America's 600,000 physicians, its wealth—as seen through its campaign contributions—makes it very influential in Washington and in state capitals. However, I predict it won't be long before drug manufacturers shift their ad dollars away from the AMA, too. I mean, if I were looking for the most bang for my advertising dollar, I'd rather expose 250 million people to my product than the small number of doctors who read medical publications.

That means that organizations such as the AMA are going to have to replace those ad revenues somehow or become less powerful on Capitol Hill. In other words, this one seemingly small change in FDA rules regarding TV ads for prescription drugs may work itself through the medical world in surprising ways—offering consumers a lift and powerful doctor groups such as the AMA a dose of reality.

Managing Care?

I met with the vice president of human resources of one of America's largest corporations not long ago. She handles all personnel matters, including the company's health benefits program. She was pleased to report that more than 85 percent of her company's 82,000 employees have enrolled in managed care programs. I've heard similar reports about many other big companies in the last two to three years.

Does that mean we're all enthralled with managed care? Not necessarily. While polls show healthy people in health maintenance organizations, preferred provider organizations and similar plans like their programs, sicker folks don't. In other words, when we need this new breed of health care delivery the most, our satisfaction plummets.

Aha! you say. So why are so many people signing up? The answer is simple: Most consumers have no other choice! An overwhelming majority of employers are phasing out fee-for-service programs for their employees. And that's not all bad. For example, at some companies, if you enroll in a managed care plan, you pay no out-of-pocket premiums, low co-payments and no deductibles. But you also lose much of the freedom you had in choosing a doctor, hospital, therapist and, depending on your program, even a pharmacist or testing facility. You also may lose the option of seeing a specialist without having prior approval by the managed care company.

Employers like managed care because it saves them money. There is no question: Companies with large groups of employees in managed care have seen their health premiums decline slightly or remain stable since 1994. However, as of 1998, premiums are starting to creep up. That's much better than the late 1980s and early 1990s, when premium costs were increasing 12 to 14 percent a year.

So if this new system is saving everyone money, maybe losing the freedom to go to any doctor we choose is worth it, even if most of us haven't exactly "chosen" managed care. Especially if health care quality is better at an HMO, as some suggest.

But is it? A 1996 study comparing managed care programs to fee-for-service plans found no significant difference in quality. In addition, no managed care company has been able to demonstrate that its doctors or hospitals get better results than the other doctors and hospitals in town.

What about prevention? A hallmark of managed care is its supposed emphasis on screening and prevention. Most companies tout their high levels of childhood immunizations and mammograms. But even these claims are somewhat deceptive. Most employers who moved their workforces to managed care already provided immunizations and mammograms as part of their previous health insurance.

And we have yet to see studies that show managed care companies perform fewer unnecessary surgeries or tests.

Don't get the idea I am against managed care. I'm actually not. Indeed, our system needs management. But so far, all that managed care has demonstrated is that it can manage discounts for big company payers. Now it must prove that it can truly improve care. If it can, we should embrace it. If it can't, we'd better have another idea.

Consumer
Power

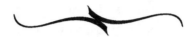

The hottest thing in medicine right now is—*you.*

That's right. Not wonder drugs or breakthrough medical surgery. No, for the first time in recent memory, everyone in the health care business is focusing on the consumer.

Pharmaceutical companies are directing their advertising at consumers. Physicians are attending conferences on how to attract and retain patients. And big insurance companies, trying to survive in the new managed care era, are wooing consumers to their health maintenance organizations with everything from free eyeglasses to discount hearing aids.

You see, without patients and the money attached to them, the health care industry is lost. And right now, the industry has more medications, more doctors, more hospitals and more HMOs than it knows what to do with.

This creates a classic supply-and-demand dynamic, one that potentially puts today's consumer in the driver's seat. But are we talking true power here, or just the illusion of it?

The answer is beginning to emerge in some new studies.

For example, one study found that 35 percent of hospital patients chose their own hospitals in 1994. Ten years earlier, only 5 percent of the public had a say about which hospital they'd use. This finding has shocked the industry. Now consumers are having more of a say. As evidence, consider how much more advertising hospitals are doing these days.

Even newer studies are showing that consumers aren't terribly impressed by HMO pitches or promotions. Instead, people choose health plans based on the listed doctors and hospitals. No matter what the HMO says about cost, quality or convenience, consumers choose the plans that have the doctors and hospitals they use and trust. This is forcing HMOs and managed care plans everywhere in the country to expand their lists of affiliated or approved providers.

In other words—and this may surprise you—managed care is providing most consumers with a wider choice of doctors and hospitals than ever before.

But probably the greatest sign of growing consumer power was revealed in December 1997. Researchers at the University of Missouri's School of Medicine found that when information about how well hospitals perform specific procedures is made public, not only do consumers make better choices but also the hospitals themselves get better. In fact, the study noted that within a year of the publication of the information, half of the Missouri hospitals studied actually added programs that improved the quality of their care.

This is truly a breakthrough finding. While the public disclosure of hospital and physician data is a growing national trend, many health experts have questioned the impact, often implying that consumers rarely use this information.

Well, clearly these "experts" are wrong. Not only are consumers using their economic clout, but they're also being empowered by the information they receive. And as a result of both, the health care market is changing.

So we consumers are hot right now, and I predict we're only going to get hotter. That's the best news I've heard in a long time.

About the Author

Charles B. Inlander is president of the People's Medical Society. As chief executive officer since its founding in early 1983, Inlander has guided the People's Medical Society to its status as the largest consumer health advocacy organization in the United States. He is also a faculty lecturer at the Yale University School of Medicine and a health commentator on Public Radio International's *Marketplace,* heard throughout the country.

He is the coauthor of many best-selling books, including *Take This Book to the Hospital With You* and *Medicine on Trial.*